C000154111

PALEO DIET

COOKBOOK

---

120 Delicious Low Carb and Healthy Recipes

for Weight Loss & Long-Term Healing

Tess Connors

Table of Contents:

INTRODUCTION

The Paleo diet is called the "stone age diet".

It is based on the presumed eating habits of our ancestors. The basic idea is: **the diet that has contributed in a fundamental way to the development and survival of man can only be good for us**.

More than forbidden or allowed foods, it is about preferring the foods that theoretically were available in the Paleolithic era.

For this reason, many dishes are naturally low carb and have a high protein content. In addition to vegetables, fruits, and other plant sources, the Paleo diet uses healthy fats instead of carbohydrates as the main protein sources.

Ready-made, highly processed foods, sweets, and fast food are avoided. To follow a Paleo diet though, you don't have to have a vegetable garden or go hunting, you can find all the foods at the supermarket (organic and otherwise). It sounds harder than it is!

The list of paleo foods is long. It includes all vegetables, nuts, fresh and dried fruits, fish, and meat.

The paleo diet has many advantages, especially when compared to a diet rich in grains and sweets. Classic foods that contain many calories and no useful substances for the body are replaced by fresh and unprocessed foods that contain many important vitamins and other nutrients.

Fast food and fried foods are outdated. After the meal, thanks to fresh foods, you will feel fit and full of energy instead of weighed down and sluggish.

Classic desserts with lots of sugar and calories, which cause the famous hunger attacks, are taboo. Instead, you can eat fiber-rich snacks that give a sense of satiety **for a long time**.

And the best thing is: paleo foods taste great. Whether it's the main course or a dessert, paleo dishes are tasty and varied; in fact, you can prepare fresh vegetables and meat in so many different ways.

By eating paleo, you will not automatically lose weight. To lose weight in the long run, you need to consume fewer calories in your daily diet than your body burns.

This cookbook will give you many ideas for Paleo-specific recipes. Enjoy, taste, and even make minor changes to the dishes if you want!

Happy reading!

MEASUREMENT CONVERSION

Volume Equivalents (Liquid)

Type	US Standard (ounces)	Metric
2 tablespoons	1 fl. oz.	30 mL
¼ cup	2 fl. oz.	60 mL
½ cup	4 fl. oz.	120 mL
1 cup	8 fl. oz.	240mL

Volume Equivalents (Dry)

Type	Metric
¼ teaspoon	1 mL
½ teaspoon	2 mL
1 teaspoon	5 mL
1 tablespoon	15 mL
¼ cup	59 mL
½ cup	118 mL
1 cup	235 mL

Oven Temperatures

Fahrenheit (°F)	Celsius (°C)
250	120
300	150
325	165
350	180
375	190
400	200
425	220
450	230

The 10 golden rules

1. Keep 10 Paleo foods on hand at all times, in your office, in your home, in your car, in your wallet. Nuts and pumpkin seeds are great options.

2. Plan a menu of meals for the week. This will help you know what to buy at the grocery store and ensure you have a delicious, healthy meal every day.

3. Cook large portions. This will help you have ready, healthy food on hand for a couple of days.

4. Don't keep foods in the house that are not paleo friendly. If this will be on hand, it will be a great temptation.

5. If you find it hard to eliminate some foods that you have a sweet tooth for that aren't 100% paleo, start decreasing the portions.

6. Don't run out of food. Can't cook anything? Don't have anything paleo at home to eat that's healthy? Are you hungry? Don't let this happen to you, it's very easy in these cases to give in to temptation.

7. Try new ingredients and seasonings. Seasonings are great for improving the taste of a dish and trying new innovative dishes.

8. If possible, freeze some of the foods you've cooked. This way, you have something on hand in the freezer, so if you don't have time to go grocery shopping, you won't starve.

9. Fall in love with plants, which are essential to your health and fitness. Don't be afraid to try new vegetables in different colors.

10. Avoid cooking the same things over and over again, you'll end up bored with your diet.

Enjoy the paleo diet and all your meals!

GROUND TURKEY WITH CABBAGE

Serv: 4 | **Prep:** 10mins | **Cook:** 40mins

Ingredients:

- ✓ 1 pound ground turkey
- ✓ 1 tablespoon of olive oil
- ✓ 1/2 tablespoon onion, diced
- ✓ 2 garlic cloves, minced
- ✓ 1 can of diced tomatoes
- ✓ 1 can of tomato sauce
- ✓ 1 tablespoon of seasoning
- ✓ 1 teaspoon of basil
- ✓ 1 teaspoon of red pepper
- ✓ salt and ground black pepper to taste
- ✓ 1 head of cabbage, cut into 1-inch squares

Directions: Place the large skillet over medium-high heat. Stir in ground turkey and cook for 5-7 minutes until crumbled and browned. Drain ground turkey and discard excess fat. Place the cooked turkey in the bowl.

Place the olive oil in a skillet and heat it over medium heat. Fry the onion in the hot oil for 5 minutes until translucent. Add the garlic to the onion and sauté for 1 minute until fragrant.

Pour in the tomato sauce and diced tomatoes. Season the mixture with red pepper, black pepper, salt, seasoning and basil. Adjust the heat to medium-low. Simmer the mixture for 10 minutes until the tomatoes are softened.

Add the cabbage. Cook for 20-25 minutes until the cabbage is tender.

Stir in ground turkey. Cook for 1-2 minutes to warm turkey.

PUMPKIN QUICHE

Serv: 6 | **Prep:** 15mins | **Cook:** 80mins

Ingredients:

- ✓ 2 pumpkins
- ✓ 1 red onion, chopped
- ✓ 1 cup chopped cooked turkey
- ✓ 4 eggs
- ✓ 1 tablespoon pumpkin pie spice
- ✓ salt to taste

Directions: Preheat oven to 175°C/350°F; on a baking sheet, place pumpkin. Grease the cake pan.

In preheated oven, bake pumpkin for 45-60 minutes until easily pierced with a fork. Cool pumpkin for 15 minutes until touchable. Halve; remove seeds. Scoop the flesh into a bowl.

Mix salt, pumpkin pie spice, eggs, turkey, onion and pumpkin until smooth in a bowl; place in prepared cake pan. In oven, bake for 35-45 minutes until center is set and edges are lighter in color.

SIRLOIN STEAK WITH LIME SAUCE AND PEPPERS

Serv: 4 | **Prep:** 15mins | **Cook:** 12

Ingredients:

- ✓ 1 lime, squeezed
- ✓ 1 tablespoon chopped garlic
- ✓ 1 teaspoon of dried oregano
- ✓ 1 teaspoon of ground cumin
- ✓ 2 tablespoons of finely chopped peppers
- ✓ bell pepper sauce
- ✓ 4 sirloin steaks (8 oz)
- ✓ salt and pepper to taste

Directions: Combine cumin, oregano, garlic and lime juice in a small bowl. Stir in peppers; use sauce to season.

Use a sharp knife to prick both sides of the meat, sprinkle with pepper and salt and transfer to a glass plate. Pour lime sauce over meat, turning to coat. Cover and refrigerate to marinate for 1 to 2 hours.

Set the grill to high heat to preheat.

Lightly grease grill with oil. Lay steaks on grill; discard marinade. Grill steaks until they reach desired doneness, or for about 6 minutes per side.

PUMPKIN STUFFED WITH APPLES AND SAUSAGES

Serv: 12 | **Prep:** 20mins | **Cook:** 1 hours

Ingredients:

- ✓ 2 pumpkins
- ✓ 2 large apples, cut into cubes
- ✓ 1 cup of pork sausage
- ✓ 1/2 onion, diced
- ✓ 1 cup of raisins
- ✓ 1/8 teaspoon of poultry seasoning
- ✓ 1/8 teaspoon ground ginger
- ✓ 1/8 teaspoon ground cloves
- ✓ 1/8 teaspoon celery seeds
- ✓ salt and ground black pepper to taste

Directions: Preheat oven to 175°C/350°F; place squash on baking sheet, cut side down.

In preheated oven, bake for 30 minutes until golden brown and soft.

Mix pepper, salt, celery seed, cloves, ginger, relish, raisins, onion, sausage and apples in a bowl; in pumpkin cavity, place sausage mixture. Place on a baking sheet. In preheated oven, bake for 30 minutes until apples are soft and sausage is cooked through.

TURKEY STUFFED WITH APPLES

Serv: 15 | **Prep:** 30 mins | **Cook:** 2h30mins

Ingredients:

- ✓ 1 whole turkey (12 pounds) - thawed, without neck and giblets
- ✓ 1/4 cup vegetable oil, or as needed
- ✓ 5 apples, core removed and cut into quarters
- ✓ 5 pounds of whole, unpeeled apples

Directions: Preheat the oven to 190°C or 375°F. If necessary, untie the legs of the turkey. Wash and use paper towels to dry the turkey. In the lidded roasting pan, place the turkey and massage the entire turkey with oil, inside and out. With apple quarters, fill neck and body cavities of turkey; in baking dish, place whole apples around turkey. In the baking dish, scatter the excess apple quarters. Place lid on baking sheet.

In prepared oven, roast for 2 1/2 to 3 hours until meat begins to separate from legs and skin turns golden brown. Uncover during the last 20 minutes of roasting, if necessary, to brown the skin. Use cooking residue for gravy, if desired.

AVOCADO BAKED EGGS

Serv: 2 | **Prep:** 10mins | **Cook:** 15mins

Ingredients:

- ✓ 1 avocado, split in half and pitted
- ✓ 2 eggs
- ✓ salt and ground black pepper to taste
- ✓ 1 pinch of cayenne pepper
- ✓ 1/4 cup of crumbled cooked bacon
- ✓ 1 tablespoon chopped fresh chives

Directions: Prepare the oven by preheating it to 425°F (220°C).

In a ramekin, place each avocado half. Crack 1 egg into each avocado half; add cayenne pepper, black pepper and salt to taste. Place ramekins on a baking sheet.

Place in the preheated oven and bake for about 15 minutes until the whole egg is cooked. Then sprinkle each avocado with chives and bacon.

RIBS WITH SPICY PAPAYA SAUCE

Serv: 4 | **Prep:** 10 mins | **Cook:** 1h50mins

Ingredients:

- ✓ 1 garlic clove, minced
- ✓ 1 cup papaya - peeled, seeded and diced
- ✓ 1/2 cup of water
- ✓ 1/2 cup white wine
- ✓ 1/2 cup of honey
- ✓ 1/4 cup of tomato paste
- ✓ 4 pounds of pork chops

Directions: In a food processor, pulse together the tomato paste, garlic, honey, papaya, wine and water for about 15 seconds, until finely chopped. In a 9-inch by 13-inch glass baking dish, place ribs with marinade; toss ribs around marinade for an even coating. Use plastic wrap to cover. Refrigerate for up to six hours or overnight.

Preheat the oven to 200°C or 400°F. Remove the ribs from the marinade and shake out the rest. Over high heat, simmer the marinade in a small saucepan. Switch to medium-low heat and simmer for 10 minutes; let rest. Place the ribs in the oven at 400°F and bake for about 1 1/2 hours until the meat can be easily pulled away from the bones. Use the reserved marinade to baste the ribs every 15 minutes.

BAKED CHICKEN BREASTS AND VEGETABLES

Serv: 4 | **Prep:** 20 mins | **Cook:** 30mins

Ingredients:

- ✓ 4 halves of chicken breast
- ✓ 8 carrots, cut into rounds
- ✓ 4 green peppers, sliced
- ✓ 8 celery stalks, chopped
- ✓ 8 green onions, chopped
- ✓ 1/4 cup chopped fresh parsley
- ✓ 1/2 cup olive oil
- ✓ 1 teaspoon salt
- ✓ 1 teaspoon of Italian seasoning
- ✓ 1 teaspoon of chili powder
- ✓ 1 teaspoon of lemon pepper
- ✓ 4 pinches of black pepper

Directions: Begin by preheating the oven to 375°F (190°C). On a baking sheet, place chicken breasts. Scatter parsley, green onion, celery, peppers and carrots around the chicken. Drizzle the vegetables and chicken with the olive oil. Season with black pepper, lemon pepper, chili powder, Italian seasoning and salt. Bake the chicken breasts in the prepared oven for half an hour or until the juices are clear and the center of the chicken breasts are no longer pink. An instant-read thermometer should register at least 165°F (74°C) when inserted into the center.

TILAPIA BAKED IN GARLIC AND OLIVE OIL

Serv: 4 | **Prep:** 5mins | **Cook:** 30mins

Ingredients:

- ✓ 4 (4 oz) Tilapia fillets

- ✓ 4 cloves of crushed garlic
- ✓ 3 tablespoons of olive oil
- ✓ 1 onion, chopped
- ✓ 1/4 teaspoon cayenne pepper

Directions: Crush the garlic, rub it on the fish fillets and place them in a shallow, non-reactive dish. Pour olive oil over the fish fillets until covered. Take some onions and place them on top of the fish. Cover the dish and place it in the fridge overnight to let the fish soak up the marinade.

Set the oven to 350°F (175°C) and begin preheating.

If using the cooking method, move the fish, onion, garlic and olive oil to a 9x13 inch baking dish. Add the white or cayenne pepper on top. If using the grill method, use aluminum foil to wrap fish with pepper, onion, garlic and oil.

Place in the oven and begin baking at 350°F (175°C) for 30 minutes.

GRILLED BEEF STEAK WITH ORANGE MARINADE

Serv: 4 | **Prep:** 15mins | **Cook:** 25mins

Ingredients:

- ✓ 2 pounds of sirloin, 2 inches thick
- ✓ 2 garlic cloves, minced
- ✓ 1 tablespoon chopped fresh ginger root
- ✓ 2 oranges, squeezed

Directions: Make cross cuts on both sides on surface of meat; transfer meat to shallow dish. Set aside 1/2 cup of the orange juice. Combine ginger, garlic and remaining orange juice. Pour mixture over meat and let marinate for a minimum of 6 hours in the refrigerator.

Turn on the grill over medium heat to preheat.

Grease grill with oil and place steak on preheated grill. Grill until cooked through for 10-12 minutes on each side. Remove the meat from the grill and let it rest for a while.

Meanwhile, heat the reserved orange juice. Cut the meat into slices and arrange on a serving platter. Drizzle the meat with the orange juice before serving.

GRILLED BEEF STEAK

Serv: 8 | **Prep:** 1mins | **Cook:** 6mins

Ingredients:

- ✓ 4 sirloin steaks (1/2 pound)
- ✓ 1/2 cup vegetable oil
- ✓ 1 ounce steak spice blend

Directions: Place the spices and oil on a plate large enough to hold the steaks. Evenly coat the steaks with the spices and oil.

Light an outdoor grill on high heat and lightly grease the grill.

Grill seasoned steaks over high heat on preheated grill until desired doneness is achieved.

GRILLED PORK CHOPS WITH GARLIC AND BASIL

Serv: 4 | **Prep:** 15 mins | **Cook:** 15mins

Ingredients:

- ✓ 4 pork chops (8 oz)
- ✓ 1 lime, squeezed
- ✓ 4 garlic cloves, minced
- ✓ 1/4 cup chopped fresh basil
- ✓ salt and black pepper to taste

Directions: In a bowl, mix lime juice and pork chops until well coated. Add the basil and garlic. Season with salt and pepper to taste. Set aside and marinate pork for 30 minutes.

Set the outdoor grill to medium heat for preheating. Lightly oil the grill.

Place the pork chops on the preheated grill and cook each side for 5-10 minutes until the center is no longer pink and the instant-read thermometer inserted into the center of the pork registers 145°F

GOAT CURRY WITH BLACK PEPPER

Serv: 4 | **Prep:** 30mins | **Cook:** 1h

Ingredients:

- ✓ 1 teaspoon of vegetable oil
- ✓ 1 onion, chopped
- ✓ 1/2 cup fresh curry leaves
- ✓ 2 tablespoons of whole black peppercorns
- ✓ 2 tablespoons of ground coriander
- ✓ 1/2 cup of water
- ✓ 3 tablespoons of vegetable oil
- ✓ 2 onions, thinly sliced
- ✓ 2 inches of ginger, chopped
- ✓ 5 cloves of garlic, minced
- ✓ 2 tablespoons of cayenne pepper, or amount as desired
- ✓ 1 tablespoon salt
- ✓ 1 tablespoon ground turmeric
- ✓ 1/2 cup of tomato paste
- ✓ 1 pound stewed goat meat, cut into 1-inch cubes
- ✓ 1/2 cup of water

Directions: In a saucepan, heat 1 teaspoon of oil over medium heat. Add the chopped onion and cook for about 7 minutes until the onion is translucent and the edges begin to brown. Transfer the onion to the blender container and set aside.

Return the saucepan to the heat and stir in the peppercorns and curry leaves. Cook, stirring, for about 5 minutes until the leaves wilt and become almost dry. Add the cilantro and cook for another 1 minute. Transfer the curry leaves to a blender and add 1/2 cup water. Blend the mixture until it forms a coarse paste.

Heat 3 tablespoons oil over medium heat in saucepan and stir in sliced onions; cook for about 5 minutes until tender and translucent. Add the garlic and ginger and continue cooking for another 3 minutes until the garlic softens. Add the turmeric, salt and cayenne pepper and cook for another 2 minutes.

Stir in the remaining 1/2 cup water, pure pepper sauce, goat meat and tomato paste. Bring the mixture to a boil, then lower the heat to medium-low, simmer with a lid on for about 30 minutes until the meat is tender.

BOB'S SWEET PEPPER SKILLET

Serv: 4| **Prep:** 15mins | **Cook:** 10mins

Ingredients:

- ✓ 2 teaspoons of extra virgin olive oil
- ✓ 2 teaspoons of sesame oil
- ✓ 3 green peppers, thinly sliced
- ✓ 1 yellow bell pepper, chopped
- ✓ 1 red bell pepper, chopped
- ✓ 1 red onion, chopped
- ✓ 2 teaspoons of minced garlic
- ✓ 1/4 teaspoon salt
- ✓ 1/4 teaspoon ground black pepper

Directions: In a large skillet, heat sesame oil and olive oil over medium heat; place pepper, salt, garlic, red onion and red, yellow and green peppers. Stir and cook bell pepper mixture for 7-10 minutes until peppers are heated through and onion is translucent.

ROAST PORK WITH CUMIN

Serv: 4| Prep: 5| Cook: 1h30mins

Ingredients:

- ✓ 3 pounds of roast pork with bone
- ✓ 2 tablespoons of dried marjoram
- ✓ salt and pepper to taste
- ✓ 3 tablespoons of cumin seeds

Directions: Preheat the oven to 165°C/325°F.

Over medium-high heat, heat roasting pan until hot. Rub pepper, salt and marjoram over roast. In the hot roasting pan, brown all sides of the roast. Sprinkle with cumin seeds. Pour in enough water to reach halfway up the sides of the roast.

Place the roast in the preheated oven, covered. Bake until internal temperature reaches 63°C/145°F for 1 1/2 hours, 30 minutes per pound. Remove from oven. Before cutting, let rest for 10 minutes.

BOPIS

Serv: 10| Prep: 15mins | Cook: 30mins

Ingredients:

- ✓ 1/2 pound of pork liver
- ✓ 1/2 pound of pork lung
- ✓ 1/2 pound of pork heart, cut into pieces
- ✓ 2 bay leaves
- ✓ 1/2 cup distilled white vinegar
- ✓ 1/2 cup of water
- ✓ salt and pepper to taste
- ✓ 3 tablespoons of olive oil
- ✓ 1 onion, chopped
- ✓ 2 garlic cloves, minced
- ✓ 2 tomatoes, diced

Directions: In two individual pots, place the pork lung and liver and add water to cover. Bring each pot to a boil; then cook for about 10 minutes until tender. Drain broth and let cool before cutting into bite-size portions. Reserve. In a large pot set over medium heat, mix the heart, lung and liver, vinegar and bay leaves. Add pepper and salt for seasoning. Bring mixture to a boil and cook for 5 minutes.

Meanwhile, in a large saucepan over medium heat, add the olive oil; cook the garlic and onion in the hot oil for about 5 minutes until fragrant. Add the tomatoes to the mixture and simmer for 5 minutes. Add the pork liver mixture from the pot into the casserole dish; stir and cook for another 5 minutes. Then serve hot.

BRAISED BEEF WITH BAROLO

Serv: 5| Prep: 30mins | Cook: 2h45mins

Ingredients:

- ✓ 1 roast beef (2 pounds)
- ✓ 1 onion, cut into 8 pieces, separate layers
- ✓ 2 large carrots, cut into 1 inch pieces
- ✓ 2 celery ribs, cut into 1-inch pieces
- ✓ 10 whole black peppercorns
- ✓ 5 whole cloves
- ✓ 1 garlic clove, crushed
- ✓ 1 cinnamon stick
- ✓ 1 sprig of rosemary
- ✓ 2 bay leaves
- ✓ 1 (750 ml) bottle of Barolo (dry red Italian wine)
- ✓ 3 tablespoons of olive oil
- ✓ 1 teaspoon salt

Directions: In a pot, put together bay leaf, rosemary, cinnamon, garlic, cloves, peppercorns, celery, carrots, onion and roast beef. Completely cover the vegetables and meat with the wine. Leave the mixture in the covered pot in the refrigerator to marinate for 6 hours. Turn the meat so that it is completely covered by the marinade on both sides; return the pot to the refrigerator and let the mixture marinate for another 6 hours.

Remove the roast beef from the marinade and place it on a plate; use paper towels to dry it well. Strain the marinade to separate the wine from the vegetable mixture. Save both the wine and the vegetable mixture.

Put the olive oil in the pot and heat it over medium-high heat. Place the beef roast and sear on all sides, each side for 4-6 minutes. Turn down to medium heat. Add the vegetable mixture. Continue to cook the beef roast for about 8 minutes, until it smells good. If there are any signs that the meat is burning, add more oil.

In the same pot, pour in the reserved wine again and salt. Lower the heat to medium-low, then cover and continue to simmer for 2 hours. Remove the lid, stir well, and continue cooking for about 10-60 minutes, until you can easily shred the meat with a fork. Remove the meat from the cooking liquid and place in a serving dish. Lay it under the foil to keep it warm.

Simmer the cooking liquid over medium-high heat until the sauce reduces consistently (about 20-30 minutes). Remove the rosemary, bay leaves, and cinnamon stick. Add the salt and use a hand-held immersion blender to blend the mixture until smooth. Finish the dish and serve by pouring the sauce over the meat.

CHICKEN CURRY IN SAUCE

Serv: 6 | **Prep:** 15mins | **Cook:** 45mins

Ingredients:

- ✓ 1 whole chicken (2 to 3 pounds)
- ✓ 1/2 teaspoon salt
- ✓ 2 tablespoons of olive oil
- ✓ 1 onion, thinly sliced
- ✓ 1/4 teaspoon ground black pepper
- ✓ 1 tablespoon crushed garlic
- ✓ 1/2 tablespoon of tomato paste
- ✓ 1/2 teaspoon of Garam Masala
- ✓ 1 teaspoon of curry powder
- ✓ 1/4 teaspoon celery salt
- ✓ 1/4 teaspoon salt
- ✓ 1/4 cup water

Directions: Begin by preheating the oven to 350°F (175°C). Place the chicken with olive oil and ½-teaspoon salt in the Dutch oven or in a 2qt. covered baking dish. Bake in the prepared oven until the chicken looks brown and is cooked through, about 40 minutes. Toss in the curry powder, Garam Masala, tomato paste, garlic, pepper, onion, seasoning to taste and 1/4 teaspoon salt. Mix it all together. Steam 1/4 cup water for the ingredients.

To blend all the flavors, return to the oven for another 5 minutes. Eat plain or enjoy with rice.

CAJUN CHICKEN

Serv: 6 | **Prep:** 30mins | **Cook:** 15mins

Ingredients:

- ✓ 1/4 cup vegetable oil
- ✓ 1/2 cup white wine
- ✓ 2 tablespoons of Cajun seasoning
- ✓ 6 halves of skinless and boneless chicken breast

Directions: Mix the Cajun seasoning, white wine and oil in a bowl. Place the chicken in the bowl and then cover it with the mixture. Cover the bowl and chill for at least three hours.

Preheat a grill over high heat.

Lightly coat the grill grate with oil. Discard the marinade and place the chicken on the grill. Let cook for about 6-8 minutes per side until the juices run clear.

MAPLE SALMON WITH CARDAMOM

Serv: 6 | **Prep:** 15mins | **Cook:** 10mins

Ingredients:

- ✓ 1 1/2 teaspoons of salt
- ✓ 1 teaspoon of paprika
- ✓ 1 teaspoon ground cardamom
- ✓ 1 teaspoon of ground coriander
- ✓ 1/2 teaspoon of ground black pepper
- ✓ 1/4 cup of grape oil
- ✓ 2 tablespoons of maple syrup
- ✓ 1 (2 pound) salmon fillet, cut into 3 inch pieces

Directions: In a bowl, mix black pepper, cilantro, cardamom, paprika and salt. Pour in maple syrup and oil and whisk until evenly combined.

Preheat nonstick skillet over medium-high heat, about 350°F (175°C).

Dip the salmon pieces into the maple syrup mixture until all sides are evenly coated.

Cook the salmon in the preheated skillet for 5-7 minutes on each side or until the fish flakes easily with a fork.

SAUSAGE MEATBALLS

Serv: 6 | **Prep:** 15mins | **Cook:** 10mins

Ingredients:

- ✓ 1 pound of ground pork shoulder
- ✓ 2 teaspoons of fennel seeds
- ✓ 2 teaspoons of fresh grated orange peel
- ✓ 1 teaspoon Kosher salt
- ✓ 1/2 teaspoon freshly ground black pepper
- ✓ 1/2 teaspoon of dried Italian herb seasoning
- ✓ 1/8 teaspoon of red pepper
- ✓ 1 pinch of grated nutmeg

Directions: Use a fork to stir in the nutmeg, red pepper, Italian seasoning, black pepper, salt, orange zest, fennel seeds and pork. Cover and refrigerate overnight.

Use plastic wrap to cover cutting board. Divide everything into 6 even pieces; roll into balls. Use plastic wrap to wrap each ball. Press plate into patties; discard plastic wrap.

Place a heavy skillet such as a cast-iron skillet over medium-high heat; in the hot skillet, cook the meatballs for 3 minutes per side until the sausage is browned and the meat is no longer pink in the center. Serve immediately.

PORK WITH CHERRY JALAPENO

Serv: 8 | **Prep:** 20mins | **Cook:** 1h

Ingredients:

- ✓ 2 pounds of boneless pork ribs, cut into pieces
- ✓ 1 tablespoon of olive oil
- ✓ 1 onion, chopped
- ✓ 1 large green bell pepper, chopped
- ✓ 1 bunch of green onions, chopped

- ✓ 1 Jalapeno bell pepper, chopped
- ✓ 4 large garlic cloves, minced
- ✓ 1 1/2 cups fresh sweet cherries, pitted and cut into quarters
- ✓ 2 tablespoons fresh coriander chopped
- ✓ 1 lime, squeezed
- ✓ 1 teaspoon of chili powder
- ✓ 1/2 teaspoon of cumin
- ✓ 1/4 teaspoon of onion powder
- ✓ 3 spoons of honey
- ✓ salt and pepper to taste

Directions: In a large saucepan covered with a lid, heat the olive oil to medium, then stir and cook the garlic, Jalapeno bell pepper, green onions, and green bell pepper for 10 minutes until soft.

Stir in onion powder, cumin, chili powder, limejuice, cilantro, cherries and pork. Bring the mixture to a boil, put a lid on and lower the heat to a simmer, then cook for half an hour until the cherries and vegetables release their juices and the pork is cooked through and no longer pink.

Remove lid, add honey and stir, then sprinkle with pepper and salt to taste. Allow to simmer without a lid for half an hour until the pork becomes tender and the sauce reduces. The sauce will not become extremely thick.

CHICKEN WITH OREGANO

Serv: 7 | **Prep:** 15mins | **Cook:** 35mins

Ingredients:

- ✓ 7 chicken legs
- ✓ 2 teaspoons of dried oregano
- ✓ salt and pepper to taste
- ✓ 1/4 cup olive oil
- ✓ 1/2 lemon, squeezed

Directions: Begin by preheating the oven to 450°F (230°C).

Rinse chicken well and pat dry. Combine pepper, salt and oregano to taste. Rub well over all chicken pieces. Arrange the chicken in a greased baking dish.

Mix lemon juice and oil; sprinkle half of mixture over chicken. Bake in the prepared oven for 15 minutes. Turn chicken pieces over and drizzle with remaining oil and lemon mixture. Bake for an additional 15 to 20 minutes. Enjoy at room temperature, cold or warm.

CHICKEN AND GARLIC STEW

Serv: 6 | **Prep:** 25mins | **Cook:** 1h15mins

Ingredients:

- ✓ 3 tablespoons of olive oil
- ✓ 5 garlic cloves, peeled
- ✓ 6 chicken thighs, halved
- ✓ 1/2 cup fresh chopped parsley
- ✓ 1/2 cup chopped celery
- ✓ 1 teaspoon of dried tarragon
- ✓ 1 tablespoon salt
- ✓ 1 teaspoon of ground white pepper
- ✓ 1/2 teaspoon of ground allspice
- ✓ 1/4 teaspoon ground cinnamon
- ✓ 1 1/2 cups of white wine

Directions: Preheat an oven to 190°C/375°F.

Place olive oil in a heavy Dutch oven that can be tightly covered. Place dry white wine, cinnamon, allspice, white pepper, salt, tarragon, celery leaves, parsley, garlic and 1/3 cup chicken; stir. Repeat twice.

Cover pan tightly; place in preheated oven. Bake for about 1 1/4 hours. Chicken will be succulent and moist but not brown; serve with crusty bread, if desired, to soak up sauce.

CLAMATO® SALMON WITH LIME

Serv: 4| **Prep:** 15mins | **Cook:** 20mins

Ingredients:

- ✓ 3 tablespoons of olive oil
- ✓ 1 medium red onion, diced
- ✓ 2 garlic cloves, sliced
- ✓ 1 fresh jalapeno pepper, seeds removed and chopped
- ✓ 1/2 bunch of cilantro, finely chopped
- ✓ 1/2 bunch of basil, finely chopped
- ✓ 2 limes, squeezed
- ✓ 1 1/2 cups of Clamato® Tomato Cocktail
- ✓ Salt and pepper to taste
- ✓ 4 salmon fillets

Directions: In a large skillet, heat olive oil over medium-high heat. Toss in the basil, cilantro, garlic, Jalapeno and onions. Then cook for 3-5 minutes. Toss in Clamato(R) and lime juice; bring to a boil. Lower heat; simmer slowly, covered.

Add pepper and salt to salmon fillets to taste, transfer to Clamato(R) broth; cook fillets for 9-12 minutes. Taste with vegetables and white rice.

SPICY CORNISH HENS

Serv: 4| **Prep:** 15mins | **Cook:** 45mins

Ingredients:

- ✓ 4 Cornish Hens
- ✓ 2 limes, halved
- ✓ 2 teaspoons of olive oil
- ✓ 1/4 teaspoon of chili powder
- ✓ 1/4 teaspoon ground cumin
- ✓ Kosher salt to taste

- ✓ ground black pepper to taste

Directions: Turn on the oven to 425°F (220°C) to preheat it.

Rub half of a lime over each hen. Drizzle hens with olive oil and season with pepper, Kosher salt, cumin and chili powder. On a rack in a shallow baking dish, place the hens.

In the preheated oven, roast the chickens for 15 minutes. Lower the heat to 350°F (175°C) and continue roasting until the internal temperature is 180°F (80°C), or about 30 minutes.

COTTAGE CHEESE CAKE WITH CABBAGE AND CAULIFLOWER

Serv: 4| **Prep:** 20mins | **Cook:** 30mins

Ingredients:

- ✓ 1 head of cauliflower, chopped
- ✓ 1/2 cup of almond milk
- ✓ 1/4 cup chopped cabbage
- ✓ 1 teaspoon ground nutmeg
- ✓ 1 pound lean ground beef
- ✓ 1 1/4 cup fresh sliced mushrooms
- ✓ 2 leeks, chopped
- ✓ 2 carrots, chopped
- ✓ 1/2 red onion, chopped
- ✓ 1 garlic clove, minced
- ✓ 1/4 cup chopped fresh cilantro

Directions: In a pot of boiling water, place cauliflower, simmer over medium heat about 15 minutes, until softened. Strain; place in the bowl of a food processor. Include nutmeg, kale and almond milk; blend until smooth.

Place the oven rack about 6 inches from the heat; preheat the oven rack.

In a skillet over medium-high heat, stir together garlic, red onion, carrots, leeks, mushrooms and ground beef; cook for 5-7 minutes, until vegetables are soft and ground beef is crumbly and brown. Spread in the bottom of an 8-inch baking dish. Transfer pureed cauliflower mixture over top.

Bake for about 10 minutes in the preheated oven, until golden brown. Garnish with fresh cilantro.

CRISPY CHICKEN WITH ONION

Serv: 4 | **Prep:** 10mins | **Cook:** 20mins

Ingredients:

- ✓ 1 pound chicken breast skinless and boned in half
- ✓ 1 1/3 cup fried onions, mashed
- ✓ 1 egg, beaten

Directions: Set the oven to 200°C or 400°F to preheat.

In a shallow bowl, scatter the crushed onions and pour the beaten egg into another shallow bowl.

Dip the chicken in the beaten egg, and then press it into the crushed onion. Gently tap the chicken to drop any loose pieces. On a baking sheet, arrange the breaded chicken.

Bake the chicken for 20 minutes, until the juices are clear and the chicken is no longer pink in the center. An instant-read thermometer should read at least 74°C or 165°F after being inserted into the center.

CUBAN PIG

Serv: 4 | **Prep:** 15mins | **Cook:** 15mins

Ingredients:

- ✓ 1 pork fillet, cut into 8 slices
- ✓ 1 lime, peeled and squeezed

- ✓ 1 teaspoon of olive oil
- ✓ 1 teaspoon of ground cumin
- ✓ 1/2 teaspoon salt
- ✓ 1 pinch of red pepper
- ✓ 1 garlic clove, pressed

Directions: Lightly flatten the pork tenderloin slices and reserve them. Combine the garlic, lime zest, crushed red pepper, olive oil, salt and cumin in a bowl. Set the limejuice aside. Brush the seasoning mixture onto each side of the pork slices.

Use cooking spray to spray a heavy skillet or rimmed grill pan and then place it over medium heat. Fry the pork slices in the pan for 6-7 minutes on each side, until golden brown on each side. Once the meat is flipped, drizzle the reserved limejuice over the meat and continue to cook until no pink color remains in the center. Serve while still hot, adding the pan juice on top.

LAMB WITH MUSHROOMS AND BACON

Serv: 4 | **Prep:** 20mins | **Cook:** 40mins

Ingredients:

- ✓ 4 lamb chops
- ✓ 2 tablespoons of olive oil
- ✓ 8 ounces of fresh sliced mushrooms
- ✓ 8 slices of bacon
- ✓ 1 teaspoon of cracked black peppercorns
- ✓ seasoned salt to taste

Directions: Prepare grill by preheating over high heat.

While the grill is heating up, place a large skillet on the stove and put in the olive oil. Put in the mushrooms; then stir and cook until softened. Reserve. Use the pepper to season the bacon slices and place them on the grill. Cook bacon until crispy, turning once, and then reserve.

Salt lamb chops to taste and place on grill. Cook to desired degree of doneness, 3 minutes per side for medium.

Present each chop with two slices of bacon and sliced mushrooms on top.

HOME CHIRPS

Serv: 12| **Prep:** 2 hours | **Cook:** 6 hours

Ingredients:

- ✓ 10 pounds of cleaned and frozen chitterlings, thawed
- ✓ 1 onion, coarsely chopped
- ✓ 2 teaspoons of salt
- ✓ 1 teaspoon of red pepper
- ✓ 1 teaspoon of minced garlic

Directions: In cold water, soak the chitterlings throughout the cleaning process. Each chitterling should be checked and run under cold water, any foreign material should be discarded and removed. The chitterlings should retain some fat, so be careful to leave some behind. Soak the chitterlings for a few minutes in 2 cold-water baths, after each has been cleaned. The second water should be clearer. Dip in 1 more bath if it is not clear.

In a 6-quart pot, place cucumbers, then add cold water until full. Bring to a boil. Put in the onion. Add red pepper flakes, garlic and salt for seasoning. Make sure that before putting in seasonings, the water is at full boil; otherwise, the cucumbers may be hard. Continue to simmer for 3-4 hours, depending on desired tenderness. Enjoy with turnip greens or spaghetti. Be sure to pass on the hot sauce and vinegar.

EASY BAKED CHICKEN THIGHS

Serv: 4| **Prep:** 5mins | **Cook:** 30mins

Ingredients:

- ✓ 4 chicken legs
- ✓ 4 teaspoons of garlic powder
- ✓ 4 teaspoons of onion flakes

Directions: Set the oven to 190°C or 375°F to preheat.

In a baking dish, arrange the thighs. Use onion flakes and garlic powder to season all sides of the chicken thighs.

In the preheated oven, bake for half an hour, until the juices are clear and the chicken is no longer pink to the bone. An instant-read thermometer should reach 74°C or 165°F after being inserted into the thickest part of the thigh near the bone.

GRILLED LOBSTER TAIL EASY

Serv: 2| **Prep:** 10mins | **Cook:** 10mins

Ingredients:

- ✓ 2 frozen lobster tails
- ✓ 1 tablespoon of olive oil
- ✓ 1 teaspoon lemon and pepper

Directions: Start by preheating the oven rack.

Partially thaw the lobster tails and cut the shells lengthwise to the back with kitchen scissors. Brush olive oil over the bare flesh and use lemon pepper for seasoning. Place on a grill pan with the open side up.

Place the pan in the oven, 6 inches from the heat source and bake for about 10 minutes until opaque and light brown at the edges.

VENISON WITH BELL PEPPER

Serv: 4| **Prep:** 15mins | **Cook:** 1h15mins

Ingredients:

- ✓ 1 pound of cubed lean venison
- ✓ 1 teaspoon salt
- ✓ 1/4 teaspoon ground black pepper
- ✓ 1 teaspoon of minced garlic
- ✓ 4 slices of onion
- ✓ 1 tablespoon chopped green bell pepper

Directions: In a large bowl, place venison. Sprinkle with garlic, pepper and salt; stir until combined. Place venison in jar with bell bell pepper and onion. Seal with ring and lid.

In the pressure canner filled with water following the manufacturer's directions, place the canner. Attach the lid. Boil with the pressure valve open. Before closing the pressure valve, boil for 5 minutes. Increase pressure to 10 psi. Lower heat to maintain pressure. Process, watching the gauge carefully so that the pressure remains at 10 psi, for 75 minutes. Turn off the heat after 75 minutes. Allow the canner to cool until the gauge reads 0 psi.

When the pressure subsides and the jar is safe to open, place the jar on a rack to cool. As it cools, the jar will close with a pop. Refrigerate the jar if it does not seal. You can store properly sealed jars in a cool, dark area.

KULAMBU EGG

Serv: 8| **Prep:** 20mins | **Cook:** 20mins

Ingredients:

- ✓ 2 tablespoons of coconut oil
- ✓ 1 large onion, chopped

- ✓ 1 tomato, chopped
- ✓ 2 teaspoons of ground cardamom
- ✓ 2 teaspoons of ground coriander
- ✓ 1 1/2 teaspoons ground cinnamon
- ✓ 1 teaspoon chopped fresh ginger root
- ✓ 1 teaspoon fresh minced garlic
- ✓ 1 teaspoon of ground cloves
- ✓ 1 teaspoon of curry powder
- ✓ 1/2 teaspoon of chili powder
- ✓ 1/2 teaspoon ground turmeric
- ✓ 1/2 teaspoon ground cumin
- ✓ 1 cup of coconut milk
- ✓ salt to taste
- ✓ 10 hard-boiled eggs, peeled and split in half lengthwise

Directions: In a saucepan, melt coconut oil over medium heat. Cook and stir tomato, onion, cilantro, cardamom, ginger, cinnamon, cloves, garlic, chili powder, curry powder, cumin and turmeric in the hot oil for about 10 minutes until onions are soft. Remove from heat and cool briefly.

In a food processor, pour in the onion mixture; remember to pulse a couple of times before letting the mixture run. Puree in batches until smooth.

Return the onion puree to the same pot; put in the coconut milk. Add salt to season mixture to taste, bring to a boil, turn down to low heat and simmer for about 5 minutes until flavors combine. Add eggs; cook for another 5 minutes until eggs are heated through.

ITALIAN CHICKEN

Serv: 8| **Prep:** 20mins | **Cook:** 45mins

Ingredients:

- ✓ 8 chicken legs
- ✓ 4 garlic cloves

- ✓ 1 tablespoon of crushed red pepper flakes
- ✓ 1 tablespoon of vegetable oil
- ✓ salt to taste
- ✓ 1/2 cup of water

Directions: Brown chicken pieces in oil in a large skillet; cook over medium heat for 15 minutes.

Crush garlic cloves; squeeze over chicken and cover pan. Cook, 10 minutes per side, over low heat. Uncover. Sprinkle with salt and red pepper flakes to taste; add water. Simmer until chicken pieces are sticky and water evaporates.

LEMON CHICKEN

Serv: 5 | **Prep:** 15mins | **Cook:** 1h

Ingredients:

- ✓ 1 whole chicken, cut into pieces
- ✓ 4 lemons, halved
- ✓ 6 garlic cloves, minced
- ✓ 1 tablespoon curry powder
- ✓ salt and pepper to taste

Directions: Set the oven to 175°C (or 350°F) and begin preheating. Place the chicken pieces in a baking dish. Squeeze the juice from the lemon halves over the chicken, then add pepper, salt, curry and garlic to taste. Bake for 60 minutes at 175°C (or 350°F) until chicken is heated through and juices are clear.

ENOKI PROTEIN EGG CAKES

Serv: 12 | **Prep:** 25mins | **Cook:** 30mins

Ingredients:

- ✓ 1 bunch of Enoki mushrooms, cut off the stem and separated
- ✓ 2 tablespoons of garlic salt
- ✓ 2 tablespoons of safflower oil

- ✓ 1/2 large shallot, chopped
- ✓ 2 garlic cloves, minced
- ✓ 1 pound ground turkey breast
- ✓ 2 yellow peppers, finely chopped
- ✓ 12 eggs
- ✓ 2 tablespoons of Italian seasoning
- ✓ salt and ground black pepper to taste

Directions: Preheat the oven to 300°F (150°C). Cough up the Enoki mushrooms with the garlic salt in a large dish. Heat oil in a large wok or skillet. Place Enoki mushrooms; cook and blend for 2-3 minutes until firm and lightly browned on the bottom. Return to plate. Place garlic and shallots in skillet; cook and blend for 1-2 minutes until fragrant. Toss with mushrooms.

Whisk the turkey into the skillet. Cook, whisking to crumble any lumps, for about 5 minutes until golden brown. Mix turkey with mushroom mixture; chop finely. Blend yellow peppers.

Whisk together the pepper, salt, Italian seasoning and eggs in a large bowl. Whisk turkey mixture together and add to two 1/3 cup muffin pans. Bake in preheated oven for about 20 minutes until edges turn brown and a toothpick inserted in the center comes out clean.

LAYERED LAMB WITH CABBAGE

Serv: 4 | **Prep:** 2hmins | **Cook:** 2h

Ingredients:

- ✓ 8 ounces of sliced lamb meat
- ✓ 1 head of cabbage, sliced and cored
- ✓ 2 cups of water
- ✓ whole black peppercorns
- ✓ salt to taste

Directions: Place a layer of sliced lamb in pot. Place a layer of cabbage on top. Repeat layer as many times as possible.

Tie in peppercorns and place in the center of the casserole. Place water over all, and put lid on to cover. Bring to a boil, and then simmer for 2 hours over low heat.

Discard the packet of peppercorns and serve.

FISH IN GINGER AND TAMARIND SAUCE

Serv: 4 | **Prep:** 15mins | **Cook:** 30mins

Ingredients:

- ✓ 1 tablespoon of cooking oil
- ✓ 1 teaspoon of mustard seeds
- ✓ 2 tablespoons fresh chopped ginger
- ✓ 1 cup chopped onions
- ✓ 2 cups of water
- ✓ 1 tablespoon of tamarind paste
- ✓ 2 tablespoons of coriander powder
- ✓ 1/2 teaspoon of ground red pepper
- ✓ salt to taste
- ✓ 1/2 pound of cod fillets, cut into 1-inch cubes
- ✓ fresh curry leaves (optional)

Directions: In a saucepan, heat the oil over medium-high heat. In the hot oil, cook the mustard seeds until they begin to pop. Add the onion and ginger.

Cook for 5 minutes. Add the water and stir in the tamarind paste. Bring to a boil. Season with salt, chili powder and cilantro. Lower the heat to medium-low. Cook for 15 minutes, stirring occasionally.

In sauce, cook fish until fish is cooked through. Top with fresh curry leaves. Serve.

FRIED TURKEY WINGS

Serv: 2 | **Prep:** 5mins | **Cook:** 25mins

Ingredients:

- ✓ 2 turkey wings
- ✓ 1 tablespoon of seasoned salt
- ✓ 1 teaspoon of seafood seasoning
- ✓ 1 teaspoon of cayenne pepper
- ✓ 2 teaspoons of garlic powder
- ✓ 4 quarts of oil for frying

Directions: Season all sides of turkey wing pieces with garlic powder, cayenne pepper, seafood seasoning and seasoned salt. Place in a plastic bag; refrigerate for 4 hours - overnight.

Heat oil to 175°C/350°F in a large deep fryer/saucepan.

Cook turkey wings for 15 minutes in hot oil; turn wings over. Cook for 10-15 minutes until meat is no longer pink to the bone.

BEEFSTEAK WITH PEPPERS

Serv: 6 | **Prep:** 5mins | **Cook:** 10mins

Ingredients:

- ✓ 2 tablespoons of olive oil
- ✓ 2 cans of peppers
- ✓ 2 pounds of beef steak

Directions: In a blender, blend the peppers and olive oil until smooth. Spread over the steak and refrigerate to marinate overnight.

Preheat grill to medium-high heat.

CHICKEN STIR FRY

Serv: 4 | **Prep:** 15 | **Cook:** 20mins

Ingredients:

- ✓ 1 tablespoon of extra virgin olive oil
- ✓ 4 halves of skinless, boneless chicken breast - cut into strips
- ✓ 1 cup julienned carrots
- ✓ 1 small onion, chopped
- ✓ 1 cup fresh sliced mushrooms
- ✓ 1 zucchini, peeled and cut into 1-inch rounds
- ✓ 2 yellow summer squash, peeled and cut into 1-inch pieces
- ✓ 1/2 cup pecans halves
- ✓ 1 teaspoon of coarsely ground black pepper

Directions: Use oil to lightly coat the bottom of a wok or nonstick skillet. Cook, stirring, the chicken strips over medium heat until lightly browned. Add onion and carrots; cook for 3 minutes.

Add the squash, zucchini and mushrooms. Cook until squash begins to soften. Add pecans; sprinkle with pepper. Saute for 2-3 minutes. Serve.

GARLIC GRILLED SHRIMP

Serv: 4 | **Prep:** 15mins | **Cook:** 15mins

Ingredients:

- ✓ 4 skewers
- ✓ 4 garlic cloves
- ✓ Kosher salt to taste
- ✓ 1/4 cup olive oil
- ✓ 1 pound large shrimp, peeled and deveined
- ✓ 1/4 teaspoon ground black pepper, or to taste

Directions: Soak the wooden skewers for no less than 15 minutes in water.

Preheat grill to medium heat; lightly oil grill.

On a cutting board, mince the garlic. Sprinkle Kosher salt over the garlic; crush the garlic on a cutting board using the back of a large knife to make a paste.

Heat olive oil and garlic paste in a skillet over medium-low heat for 5 minutes until garlic begins to brown; remove from heat.

On each skewer, thread 5 shrimp through the top of the body and tail to skewer the shrimp. Season the shrimp with pepper and Kosher salt. Brush garlic-scented olive oil on 1 side of shrimp.

Place shrimp on preheated grill, oil side down. Brush with more olive oil; cook for 4 minutes until shrimp begin to curl and turn pink. Turn shrimp over; brush with olive oil once more. Grill for 4 minutes until shrimp are pink all over and opaque.

CHICKEN COOKED IN COCONUT MILK

Serv: | **Prep:** 20mins | **Cook:** 35mins

Ingredients:

- ✓ 3 tablespoons of oil
- ✓ 1/2 cup fresh sliced ginger
- ✓ 1 whole chicken, cut into pieces
- ✓ salt and ground black pepper to taste
- ✓ 2 cans of coconut milk
- ✓ 10 ounces of thawed chopped spinach

Directions: In a large skillet over medium heat, add the oil and stir in the ginger slices. Stir and cook until lightly browned and fragrant. Remove the ginger and reserve it. Season the chicken with pepper and salt. Place the chicken in the same skillet over medium-high heat without crowding it. Cook the chicken until all sides turn light brown. Return the ginger to the skillet and add the coconut milk. Bring to a boil and then close the pan with a tilted lid to let the steam escape. Lower the heat to medium-low and simmer for about 30 minutes until the chicken is pink to the bone, stirring occasionally.

Add the spinach. Simmer for 8-12 minutes, without a lid, until spinach is well heated through. Add pepper and salt to taste, if needed.

GRAPEFRUIT CHICKEN

Serv: 6 | **Prep:** 10mins | **Cook:** 1h

Ingredients:

- ✓ 1 whole chicken, rinsed and dried
- ✓ 1 grapefruit, cut in half
- ✓ 1 tablespoon of olive oil
- ✓ 1/2 teaspoon of seasoned salt

Directions: Set the oven to 400°F (200°C) and begin preheating.

Arrange the chicken in a baking dish; squeeze the juice from the grapefruit halves over and into the chicken. Add the olive oil on top and sprinkle with seasoned salt. Wrap with aluminum foil.

Bake for 45 minutes, covered, in the preheated oven; remove the foil and continue to bake for another 15 minutes until the chicken juices run clear and the meat loses its pink color at the bone. An instant-read thermometer inserted into the thickest part of the thigh, near the bone, should show 180°F (82°C). Remove the chicken from the oven and wrap it with 2 layers of aluminum foil; let it rest for 10 minutes in a warm area before slicing.

CAJUN GRILLED CHICKEN

Serv: 7 | **Prep:** 20mins | **Cook:** 1h

Ingredients:

- ✓ 6 halves of skinless and boneless chicken breast
- ✓ 4 links of pork sausage
- ✓ 2 Jalapeno peppers, seeded and chopped
- ✓ 3/4 cup chopped onion
- ✓ 3 garlic cloves, minced
- ✓ 1 teaspoon of Cajun seasoning
- ✓ 12 slices of bacon

Directions: Open each chicken breast. Cut each sausage in half lengthwise, and then slice to the length of the chicken breast. Place a halved sausage ring inside each chicken breast; place garlic, onion, and Jalapeno peppers for seasoning, and use toothpicks to seal the chicken. Season the outside with Cajun spices (or Cajun seasoning). Wrap each breast with 2 slices of bacon and use toothpicks to secure. Place on a barbecue grill over medium coals and grill until cooked through, about 30 minutes per side. Enjoy!

GRILLED CHICKEN AND HERBS

Serv: 4 | **Prep:** 15mins | **Cook:** 20

Ingredients:

- ✓ 4 large halves of skinless, boneless chicken breast
- ✓ 2 tablespoons of olive oil
- ✓ 1 teaspoon of dried rosemary
- ✓ 1 teaspoon of dried thyme
- ✓ 1 teaspoon of dried oregano
- ✓ 1 teaspoon of minced garlic
- ✓ 1/2 teaspoon salt
- ✓ 1/2 teaspoon of ground black pepper

Directions: Prepare the grill over medium heat and lightly coat the grill with oil.

Rinse chicken breasts, pat dry with paper towels and pierce a few times with a fork. In a large resealable plastic bag, place the chicken breasts and add the olive oil. Close the bag and shake to mix the chicken with the olive oil; add black pepper, salt, garlic, oregano, thyme and rosemary to the bag, close and shake again to mix the chicken with the herbs.

On the preheated grill, grill chicken breasts for 10 minutes per side until an instant-read meat thermometer indicates 160°F (70°C) when you insert it into the thickest section of meat and the juices run clear.

GRILLED CHICKEN WITH ROSEMARY AND BACON

Serv: 4 | **Prep:** 10mins | **Cook:** 16mins

Ingredients:

- ✓ 4 teaspoons of garlic powder
- ✓ 4 halves of skinless and boneless chicken breast
- ✓ salt and pepper to taste
- ✓ 4 sprigs of fresh rosemary
- ✓ 4 slices of thick bacon

Directions: Lightly oil the grate of an outdoor grill preheated over medium-high heat.

Sprinkle chicken breast with 1-teaspoon garlic powder; add pepper and salt for seasoning. Scatter a sprig of rosemary over the chicken breast. Wrap chicken with bacon to keep rosemary in place. Insert a toothpick or other large stalk of rosemary into the bacon to secure it.

Cook each side of the chicken breasts for 8 minutes until they are pink in the center and the juices are clear. After cooking, make sure an instant-read thermometer measures a minimum of 165°F (74°C) when inserted in the center. Stay close to the grill to extinguish any flames that arise from the bacon. Discard the toothpicks and serve.

GRILLED CHICKEN WITH COLESLAW

Serv: 6 | **Prep:** 45mins | **Cook:** 10mins

Ingredients:

For the marinade:

- ✓ 3 tablespoons of apple cider vinegar
- ✓ 3 tablespoons of molasses
- ✓ 3 tablespoons of olive oil
- ✓ 3/4 teaspoon of ground allspice
- ✓ 3/4 teaspoon salt
- ✓ 3/4 teaspoon of freshly ground black pepper
- ✓ 6 boneless and skinless chicken thighs

For the salad:

- ✓ 6 tablespoons apple cider vinegar
- ✓ 2 teaspoons of honey
- ✓ 6 slices of bacon
- ✓ 1 teaspoon of cumin seeds, lightly crushed
- ✓ 1 packet DOLE® Classic Coleslaw
- ✓ 2 large green onions DOLE

Directions: Mix together pepper, salt, and allspice, olive oil, molasses and 3 tablespoons cider vinegar.

Place chicken in a dish; pour marinade over chicken, then turn to coat. Refrigerate with a lid on for half an hour.

Remove chicken from marinade, and then put away remaining marinade. Grill until no pink meat remains in the middle, 3-4 minutes per side. Cover and keep warm.

In a bowl, mix the honey and the rest of the vinegar, and then stir.

In a large skillet, cook and stir the bacon over medium heat until crispy. Break bacon into small pieces. Reserve 2 tablespoons of bacon fat.

Bring bacon grease to medium-high heat until hot but not releasing smoke; cook and stir cumin seeds for about half a minute until aromatic.

Place pepper, salt, vinegar mixture and coleslaw to taste; cook and stir for about 60 seconds until cabbage is just wilted. Remove skillet from heat; place bacon and green onions. Combine.

Divide salad among 6 separate plates and add cooked chicken, then serve.

GROUND BEEF AND CABBAGE

Serv: 6 | **Prep:** 15mins | **Cook:** 45mins

Ingredients:

- ✓ 1 large head of cabbage, finely chopped
- ✓ 1 can of diced tomatoes with juice
- ✓ 1 onion, halved and thinly sliced
- ✓ 1 tablespoon of Italian seasoning
- ✓ salt and ground black pepper to taste
- ✓ 1 pound lean ground beef

Directions: Over low heat, mix cabbage, black pepper, tomatoes with juice, salt, onion and Italian seasoning in a large pot; let simmer.

Add the ground beef and then crumble it in. Cook for 45 minutes, covered, until beef is fully cooked and cabbage is tender. Stir occasionally.

GROUND TURKEY TACOS

Serv: 4 | **Prep:** 10mins | **Cook:** 45mins

Ingredients:

Tacos:

- ✓ 1 tablespoon of vegetable oil
- ✓ 1-pound lean ground turkey (at least 93%)
- ✓ 1 (1 ounce) packet Old El Paso® taco seasoning mix
- ✓ 2/3 cup of water
- ✓ 1 (4.6 ounce) package of Old El Paso® taco shells

Gaskets:

- ✓ 2 medium avocados, pitted, peeled and sliced
- ✓ 1 cup sliced pineapple (fresh or canned)

Directions: Heat oil in a 10-inch skillet over medium-high heat. Cook the turkey until no longer pink, and then drain.

Add the water and Tacos seasoning mixture. Lower the heat and simmer without a lid until thickened, about 5-10 minutes.

Pour the filling into the Tacos shells. Add toppings.

BEEF WITH HERBS IN SALT CRUST

Serv: 8 | **Prep:** 15mins | **Cook:** 1h

Ingredients:

- ✓ 1/3 cup olive oil
- ✓ 1/4 cup chopped onion
- ✓ 1 teaspoon of garlic salt
- ✓ 1 teaspoon of dried basil
- ✓ 1/2 teaspoon of dried marjoram
- ✓ 1/2 teaspoon of dried thyme
- ✓ 1/4 teaspoon ground black pepper

- ✓ 3 pounds of roast beef
- ✓ 3 pounds Kosher salt
- ✓ 1 1/4 cup of water

Directions: In a heavy plastic bag, mix pepper, thyme, marjoram, basil, garlic salt, onion and oil; combine properly. Include roast; coat well with marinade. Refrigerate for 2 hours or overnight to marinate.

Set the oven to 350°F (175°C) and begin preheating. Use aluminum foil to line a baking sheet.

Mix Kosher water and salt to make a thick dough. Scoop 1 cup of dough into a 1/2-inch-thick rectangle in the skillet. Use paper towels to dry roast; insert a meat thermometer. Lay roast on a layer of salt; pack remaining salt paste around meat to seal well. Bake until thermometer reads 140°, 60-70 minutes. (Steam may cause crust to crack slightly). Remove from oven; let rest for 10 minutes. Remove and discard salt crust.

PORK CHOPS WITH HERBS

Serv: 4 | **Prep:** 5mins | **Cook:** 10mins

Ingredients:

- ✓ 1/3 cup of dried parsley
- ✓ 1/4 cup dried marjoram
- ✓ 1/4 cup dried thyme
- ✓ 3 tablespoons of rubbed sage
- ✓ 2 tablespoons garlic powder
- ✓ 2 tablespoons of onion powder
- ✓ 1 teaspoon salt
- ✓ 1 teaspoon ground cinnamon
- ✓ 4 boneless pork chops
- ✓ 2 teaspoons of vegetable oil, or as desired
- ✓ 1 tablespoon oil

Directions: In a bowl, mix together cinnamon, salt, onion powder, garlic powder, sage, thyme, marjoram and parsley. Rub each pork chop with ½ teaspoon of herb mixture. Store remaining herb mixture for later use in airtight container.

In a large skillet, heat the oil over medium heat. In the skillet, cook the pork chops for 4 to 5 minutes on each side or until the center is no longer pink. The instant-read thermometer should register 145°F (63°C) when inserted in the center.

HONEY AND JALAPENO BURGER

Serv: 5 | **Prep:** 5mins | **Cook:** 15mins

Ingredients:

- ✓ 1 pound lean ground beef
- ✓ 1 1/2 spoons of honey
- ✓ 1 1/2 tablespoons of diced Jalapeno pepper

Directions: Preheat outdoor grill to medium-high heat; lightly oil grill.

Using your hands, mix honey, Jalapeno chiles and ground beef in a large bowl; form into 4 equal patties.

On preheated grill, cook 7-10 minutes per side for well done, until burgers are cooked to preferred doneness. An instant-read thermometer inserted in the center should read 70°C/160°F.

HONEY SMOKED TURKEY

Serv: 16 | **Prep:** 30mins | **Cook:** 3h15mins

Ingredients:

- ✓ 1 whole turkey
- ✓ 2 tablespoons chopped fresh sage
- ✓ 2 tablespoons of ground black pepper
- ✓ 2 tablespoons celery salt

- ✓ 2 tablespoons chopped fresh basil
- ✓ 2 tablespoons of vegetable oil
- ✓ 1 (12 oz) jar of honey
- ✓ 1/2 pound of Mesquite shavings

Directions: Prepare grill, set on high heat. Use twice the normal amount of charcoal if using a charcoal grill.

Place wood chips in a pile of water, let them soak near the grill. Prepare the turkey by removing the neck, innards and gravy packet. Rinse well in cold water and pat dry with paper towels.

Place turkey in a large disposable baking dish. Combine the vegetable oil, sage, ground black pepper, basil and celery salt in a bowl. Rub the mixture evenly all over the turkey. With the bird facing the breast in the roasting pan, cover the pan with aluminum foil.

Place a handful of soaked wood shavings in the coals, place the roasting pan on the prepared grill. Bake for 1 hour with the grill lid closed. Add 2 more handfuls of wood chips to the coals.

Pour half of the honey over the turkey and replace the aluminum foil. Continue cooking with the lid closed for 1 1/2 to 2 hours, or until the internal temperature of the thickest part of the thigh is 180°F (80°C).

Remove the aluminum foil and gently turn the turkey from the breast side up. Brush the surface with the remaining half of the honey and bake uncovered for another 15 minutes.

The cooked turkey will be very dark because of the cooked honey.

HONEY TROUT

Serv: 4 | **Prep:** 10mins | **Cook:** 15mins

Ingredients:

- ✓ 1 pound of trout fillets
- ✓ 1/3 cup honey
- ✓ 2 tablespoons of Mesquite seasoning
- ✓ 1 teaspoon of ground black pepper
- ✓ 1 teaspoon of seasoned salt

Directions: Preheat the oven to 230°C/450°F. Line a sheet of aluminum foil on a baking sheet.

Place the trout on the prepared baking sheet, skin side down. Use honey to cover the trout. Sprinkle salt, black pepper and Mesquite seasoning over the honey. Use a fork to press the seasonings and honey into the trout.

Bake in preheated oven for 15-20 minutes until fish flakes easily with a fork.

HENS WITH POPPY, HONEY AND GINGER

Serv: 4 | **Prep:** 15mins | **Cook:** 1h

Ingredients:

- ✓ 2 Rock Cornish Hens
- ✓ 1/2 teaspoon salt
- ✓ 1/2 teaspoon of ground black pepper
- ✓ 1/3 cup honey
- ✓ 1 tablespoon poppy seeds
- ✓ 1 1/2 teaspoons of mustard powder
- ✓ 3/4 teaspoon of ground ginger

Directions: Begin by preheating the oven to 350°F (175°C). Spray nonstick spray on the grill of the shallow baking pan. Cut each hen in half and arrange in the baking dish, skin side down. Sprinkle with pepper and salt.

Whisk together the ginger, mustard, poppy seeds and honey. Brush the mixture onto both sides of the chickens.

Roast uncovered, turning once, for 60 minutes.

INDIAN CAULIFLOWER

Serv: 5| **Prep:** 10mins| **Cook:** 40mins

Ingredients:

- ✓ 1 large head of cauliflower
- ✓ 4 tablespoons of vegetable oil
- ✓ 1/2 teaspoon ground turmeric
- ✓ 1 small onion, chopped
- ✓ 2 tomatoes, pureed
- ✓ 1 teaspoon garlic powder
- ✓ 3 teaspoons of Garam Masala
- ✓ salt to taste
- ✓ 1/2 head of lettuce

Directions: Set the oven to 350°F (175°C) and begin preheating. Cut off most of the stem of the cauliflower; arrange the entire head in a baking dish.

In a small skillet, heat together turmeric and 2 tablespoons oil. Brush the mixture over the head of the cauliflower. Cook the cauliflower for 30 minutes.

Meanwhile, in a skillet, heat 2 tablespoons oil; sauté chopped onions until medium brown. Add the salt, Garam Masala, garlic powder and pureed tomatoes. Simmer the mixture for 10 minutes.

Place the lettuce leaves on a serving platter. Add the cauliflower. Transfer the tomato curry to the top. Serve warm.

INDIAN CHICKEN CURRY

Serv: 6| **Prep:** 15mins | **Cook:** 30mins

Ingredients:

- ✓ 8 chicken breast halves
- ✓ 1 tablespoon of olive oil
- ✓ 2 onions, peeled and cut into quarters
- ✓ 1 teaspoon of chopped fresh ginger root
- ✓ 1 teaspoon crushed garlic
- ✓ 1 tablespoon hot curry (Madras) powder
- ✓ 1 can of tomato sauce
- ✓ 1 can of coconut milk
- ✓ 4 whole cloves
- ✓ 4 cardamom pods
- ✓ 1 cinnamon stick
- ✓ salt to taste

Directions: Rinse and dry chicken; sprinkle with pepper and salt to taste. Over medium-high heat, heat oil in a large skillet. Sauté chicken in hot oil until golden brown; remove from skillet and set aside. Fry the onions in the pan until light; put in the garlic and ginger. Fry until aromatic, then stir in curry powder. Return the chicken to the pan; add the cinnamon stick, tomato sauce, cardamom, cloves and coconut milk. Sprinkle with salt to taste then toss to combine.

Turn over low heat; simmer for 20-25 minutes until chicken is cooked through, tender and not pink inside.

INDIAN BHURTHA EGGPLANT

Serv: 4| **Prep:** 15mins | **Cook:** 50mins

Ingredients:

- ✓ 1 eggplant
- ✓ 2 tablespoons of vegetable oil
- ✓ 1/2 teaspoon of cumin seeds

- ✓ 1 medium onion, sliced
- ✓ 1 teaspoon fresh chopped ginger
- ✓ 1 large tomato - peeled, seeded and diced
- ✓ 1 garlic clove, minced
- ✓ 1/2 teaspoon ground turmeric
- ✓ 1/2 teaspoon ground cumin
- ✓ 1/2 teaspoon of ground coriander
- ✓ 1/4 teaspoon cayenne pepper
- ✓ 1/2 teaspoon salt, or to taste
- ✓ ground black pepper to taste
- ✓ 1/4 cup chopped fresh cilantro

Directions: Prepare and preheat oven rack. Brush the eggplant on the outside with oil, or coat with cooking spray. Place eggplant under grill and bake for about 30 minutes, or until tender and skin is blistered.

Turn as needed to fully cook the eggplant. Cut in half-lengthwise, scoop out the flesh from the skin, and discard the skin. Chop the eggplant flesh and set aside.

Heat the oil in a large skillet or work over medium high heat. Then add the cumin seeds, let crackle for a few seconds or until golden brown. Be careful not to burn the seeds. Add and sauté the onions, garlic and ginger until tender be careful that the onions do not get too brown.

Add the tomatoes and seasonings of ground turmeric, cumin and coriander, cayenne pepper, black pepper and salt. Continue to cook and stir for a few minutes or until cooked through.

Place the eggplant pieces in the skillet, and cook for 10-15 minutes, allowing its moisture to evaporate. Test to taste, and adjust the seasoning as desired.

Sprinkle with fresh cilantro before serving.

INSTANT POT® LEMON ROASTED CHICKEN

Serv: 6 | **Prep:** 5mins | **Cook:** 34mins

Ingredients:

- ✓ 1 whole chicken
- ✓ 1 lemon, cut
- ✓ 2 tablespoons of olive oil
- ✓ 1 teaspoon garlic powder
- ✓ 1 teaspoon of paprika
- ✓ 1/2 teaspoon of ground black pepper
- ✓ 1 cup of chicken broth
- ✓ salt

Directions: Rinse chicken with water and pat dry. Fill the cavity of the chicken with lemon wedges.

Set the multi-function pressure cooker as an Instant Pot ® in Sauté mode. In a bowl, combine pepper, olive oil, paprika, garlic powder and salt. Rub half of the mixture over the top of the chicken. Set in pot with breast side down, cook for 3-4 minutes until crispy.

Rub the remaining half of the mixture into the bottom of the chicken. Use tongs to turn and cook for another minute.

Remove the chicken from the pot. Place a trivet in the pot. Place chicken on trivet with breast side down; pour chicken broth into pot. Close lid and place on high pressure for 20 minutes as specified in the pot manual. Allow pressure to increase for 10-15 minutes.

Relieve pressure naturally for 10-40 minutes according to pot manual.

ARTICHOKES IN INSTANT POT®

Serv: 4| **Prep:** 5mins | **Cook:** 20mins

Ingredients:

- ✓ 1 cup of water
- ✓ 2 garlic cloves
- ✓ 1 bay leaf
- ✓ 1/2 teaspoon salt
- ✓ 4 artichokes, trimmed and cut
- ✓ 2 tablespoons of lemon juice

Directions: In a multi-purpose pressure cooker (such as Instant Pot®), mix water, bay leaf, garlic and salt. Place a steamer in the pot and add artichokes with the top cut side up. Pour the lemon juice over the artichokes. Seal the lid and, following the manufacturer's directions, put on high pressure and set a timer to 10 minutes. Allow pressure to increase for 10-15 minutes. Using the quick release method according to the manufacturer's directions, carefully release the pressure for 5 minutes, then unseal and remove the lid.

Cool the artichokes until they can be handled easily. One at a time, remove outer petals and pull through teeth to get the soft part of the petal. Discard any leftover petals. Pull the center out of the stem and throw it away. Cut artichokes into pieces or eat the bottom entirely.

INSTANT POT® VEGAN SPAGHETTI SQUASH WITH PESTO

Serv: 4| **Prep:** 10mins | **Cook:** 20mins

Ingredients:

Spaghetti squash:

- ✓ 1 spaghetti squash, halved and with seeds

- ✓ 1 cup of vegetable broth
- ✓ 1 sprig of fresh rosemary chopped
- ✓ 1/2 teaspoon salt

Pesto:

- ✓ 2 cups of fresh basil leaves
- ✓ 2/3 cup olive oil
- ✓ 1/4 cup pine nuts
- ✓ 2 tablespoons of nutritional yeast
- ✓ 2 garlic cloves
- ✓ 1/2 teaspoon salt
- ✓ 1/4 teaspoon ground black pepper

Directions: In a multipurpose pressure cooker such as Instant Pot, mix 1/2 teaspoon salt, rosemary, vegetable broth and squash, close lid. Lock. Following manufacturer's instructions, choose high pressure. Set timer to 7 minutes; let pressure build for 10-15 minutes.

Carefully use quick release method following manufacturer's instructions to release pressure for 5 minutes. Unlock lid; remove. Remove pumpkin; chill for 5-10 minutes until easy to handle. Use a fork to scrape inside of pumpkin into spaghetti strands.

In the bowl of a food processor, place the pepper, 1/2 teaspoon salt, garlic, nutritional yeast, pine nuts, olive oil and basil leaves until smooth. Serve over the spaghetti.

PALEO ITALIAN CHICKEN MEATLOAF

Serv: 8| **Prep:** 15mins | **Cook:** 2h

Ingredients:

- ✓ 6 carrots
- ✓ 1 celery stalk
- ✓ 1/4 big onion
- ✓ 2 garlic cloves
- ✓ 1 tablespoon of Italian seasoning

- ✓ 1 teaspoon of ground black pepper
- ✓ 7 chicken fillets
- ✓ 4 eggs
- ✓ 1 can of tomato sauce without added salt, divided

Directions: Preheat oven to 350°F (175°C). Grease 9x5-inch baking dish.

Add black pepper, Italian seasoning, garlic, onion, celery and carrots to food processor; process until vegetables are chopped. Move vegetable mixture to a large bowl.

Process the chicken fillets in a food processor until ground.

Beat eggs to vegetable mixture with fork until incorporated; put in 1/2 of the tomato sauce and stir. Fold the chicken into the tomato sauce and vegetable mixture; add to the prepared baking dish.

Bake in preheated oven for 1.5 hours; spread leftover tomato sauce over top of meatloaf. Continue baking for about half an hour until the meatloaf is fully cooked. The instant-read thermometer inserted in the center should reach no less than 165°F (74°C). Let it cool in the pan for 20 minutes before slicing.

CHICKEN CURRY JAMAICAN STYLE

Serv: 4 | **Prep:** 10mins | **Cook:** 45mins

Ingredients:

- ✓ 1/4 cup vegetable oil
- ✓ 1 onion, chopped
- ✓ 1 tomato, chopped
- ✓ 1 garlic clove, minced
- ✓ 2 tablespoons of Jamaican-style curry powder
- ✓ 2 slices of Habanero pepper (optional)
- ✓ 1/4 teaspoon of ground thyme

- ✓ 2 halves of boneless, skinless chicken breast, cut into 1-inch pieces
- ✓ 1 cup of water
- ✓ 1/2 teaspoon salt, or to taste

Directions: In a skillet, heat vegetable oil over medium-high heat; cook and stir in thyme, Habanero pepper, curry powder, garlic, tomato and onion for about 7 minutes or until onion is golden brown. Add chicken, stir and cook for about 5 minutes or until lightly browned.

Add the water to the pan, lower the heat to low; simmer, covered, for about 30 minutes or until the center of the chicken is no longer pink. Salt.

CRISPY BAKED BACON

Serv: 6 | **Prep:** 5mins | **Cook:** 15mins

Ingredients:

- ✓ 1 package of thick-cut bacon

Directions: Line up 2 sheets of aluminum foil on a large baking sheet; cover baking sheet completely. Place bacon strips on prepared baking sheet, with a minimum of 1/2 inch spacing between strips. Place baking sheet in cold oven. Heat an oven to 220°C/425°F. Allow the bacon to bake for 14 minutes. Place cooked bacon on paper towel-lined plates. To crisp up the bacon, cool for 5 minutes.

JUICY ROAST CHICKEN

Serv: 6 | **Prep:** 10mins | **Cook:** 1h15mins

Ingredients:

- ✓ 1 whole chicken
- ✓ salt and black pepper to taste
- ✓ 1 tablespoon of onion powder

- ✓ 1/2 cup margarine, divided
- ✓ 1 celery stalk, without leaves

Directions: Preheat the oven to 175°C/350°F. Place chicken in a baking dish. Season generously inside and out with pepper and salt. Sprinkle onion powder inside and out. Place 3 tablespoons margarine in the cavity of the chicken. Place some of the leftover margarine around the outside of the chicken. Cut celery into 3-4 pieces. Place in the cavity of the chicken. Bake in preheated oven, uncovered, for 1 hour and 15 minutes, to achieve at least an internal temperature of 82°C/180°F. Remove from heat. Baste with drippings and melted margarine. Use aluminum foil to cover. Let stand for about 30 minutes and then serve.

SOFT CHICKEN IN POT

Serv: 4 | **Prep:** 10mins | **Cook:** 8h

Ingredients:

- ✓ 1 pound of chicken breast
- ✓ 1 diced tomato
- ✓ 1/4 onion, chopped (optional)
- ✓ 1 teaspoon of Italian seasoning (optional)
- ✓ 1 garlic clove, minced (optional)

Directions: In a slow cooker, place the chicken, and then pour in the tomatoes. Add the garlic, Italian seasoning and onion. Cook the chicken mixture for 6-8 hours on low.

CHICKEN WITH POMEGRANATE SAUCE

Serv: 12 | **Prep:** 20mins | **Cook:** 3h30mins

Ingredients:

- ✓ 1/2 cup vegetable oil
- ✓ 4 medium red onions, thinly sliced
- ✓ 3 pounds of bone-in chicken pieces
- ✓ 2 cups of hot water or as needed
- ✓ 2 1/2 cups of pomegranate juice
- ✓ 4 cups chopped walnuts
- ✓ 2 tablespoons of freshly ground cardamom
- ✓ 2 tablespoons ground cinnamon
- ✓ 1 medium-sized pumpkin, seeded and cubed
- ✓ 1/4 teaspoon of saffron powder
- ✓ 1 teaspoon of salt, or to taste

Directions: Place the oil in a large heavy skillet and heat over medium heat. Cook and stir the sliced onion until it becomes translucent and soft, about 5 minutes. Adjust the heat to medium-low, and continue to cook and stir for another 15-20 minutes until the onion is dark brown and very tender.

Adjust heat to medium-high. Stir in chicken pieces. Fry until outside turns light brown. Pour in water and bring mixture to a boil. Adjust heat to low. Simmer for another 30 minutes, pouring in more water if the mixture begins to dry out.

Set the oven to 325°F or 65°C.

In a blender or food processor, blend the pomegranate juice and walnuts until pureed (you can do this in batches if necessary). Pour the puree into the chicken over low heat. Season the mixture with salt, saffron powder, cardamom and cinnamon. Add the cubed pumpkin. Spread the mixture into a baking dish.

Cover the dish and let it bake in the preheated oven for 2 1/2 hours. Serve together with the white rice.

32

LAMB SHANK BRAISED IN WHITE WINE WITH ROSEMARY

Serv: 4 | **Prep:** 10mins | **Cook:** 2h50mins

Ingredients:

- ✓ 3 tablespoons of olive oil
- ✓ 4 lamb shanks
- ✓ 5 garlic cloves, sliced
- ✓ 1 small onion, chopped
- ✓ 2 teaspoons chopped fresh rosemary, plus sprigs for garnish
- ✓ 1 pinch of salt and freshly ground black pepper
- ✓ 1 cup of dry white wine

Directions: Heat the oil in a large skillet over medium-high heat. Place the shanks in the hot skillet. Brown all sides for about 12 minutes. Place on a plate.

Lower the heat to medium-low. Add the garlic to the pan. Cook for 30-40 seconds. Add the onion. Sauté for 6-8 minutes and continue cooking until translucent. Place the shanks in the skillet. Season with pepper, salt to taste and 2 tablespoons fresh rosemary.

Toss in the wine. Bring the heat to medium-high. Simmer. Lower the heat to low. Simmer, tightly covered, until shanks are very tender when pricked with a knife for 2-2 1/2 hours.

Turn 1-2 times during cooking. Add water if necessary to maintain original liquid level. Garnish with sprigs of rosemary.

Serve the shanks.

CORNISH HENS ROASTED WITH LEMON LEEKS

Serv: 4 | **Prep:** 10mins | **Cook:** 1h

Ingredients:

- ✓ 4 Rock Cornish Hens
- ✓ 2 lemons, halved
- ✓ 2 sliced leeks, only the white part
- ✓ 2 tablespoons of poultry seasoning

Directions: Preheat an oven to 175°C/350°F.

Place hens in a lightly greased 9x13-inch baking dish. Use 1/4 sliced leek and 1 lemon half to stuff each hen; sprinkle with dressing.

Bake for 1 hour until juices are clear and hens cook at 175°C/350°F; rest for 10 minutes. Remove leeks and lemons.

COD WITH LEMON AND PEPPER

Serv: 4 | **Prep:** 5mins | **Cook:** 10mins

Ingredients:

- ✓ 3 tablespoons of vegetable oil
- ✓ 1 1/2 pounds of cod fillets
- ✓ 1 lemon, squeezed
- ✓ ground black pepper to taste

Directions: Set the heat to medium-high and heat the oil in a large skillet until hot. Fry the fillets and pour the juice of 1/2 lemon over the tops. Season with the pepper.

Fry for 4 minutes and then flip. Pour in the rest of the lemon juice and season with pepper.

Continue frying until the fillets flake easily with a fork.

PORK SAUSAGES

Serv: 4 | **Prep:** 15mins | **Cook:** 1h

Ingredients:

- ✓ 10 pounds of ground pork
- ✓ 2 pounds of ground pork liver
- ✓ 4 onions, chopped
- ✓ salt and pepper to taste
- ✓ 4 sausage casings

Directions: Combine pepper, salt, onions, liver and pork together. Place in casing and boil in water for 60 minutes.

CHICKEN BREAST WITH CURRY AND GINGER

Serv: 4 | **Prep:** 30mins | **Cook:** 30mins

Ingredients:

- ✓ 2 tablespoons of vegetable oil
- ✓ 1 teaspoon of cumin seeds
- ✓ 2 medium onions, finely chopped
- ✓ 1 teaspoon ground turmeric
- ✓ 1 teaspoon of cayenne pepper to taste
- ✓ 1 teaspoon of Garam Masala
- ✓ 1 garlic clove, minced
- ✓ 1 tablespoon chopped ginger
- ✓ 5 peeled tomatoes, seeds removed and cut into pieces
- ✓ 1 pound of chicken breast meat

Directions: In a large saucepan, heat the oil over medium heat. Stir in the cumin seeds and cook for 20-45 seconds until they begin to pop. Stir in onion and cook for 5 minutes until golden brown. Season with ginger, garlic, Garam Masala, cayenne and turmeric. Cook until aromatic, about 1-2 minutes.

Place the tomatoes with the mixture in a blender and puree until smooth. Transfer the puree to the saucepan and add the chicken. Bring to a gentle boil for 20 minutes until chicken is cooked; while cooking, add water if necessary to maintain preferred consistency.

EGGS AND TOMATO SAUCE

Serv: 4 | **Prep:** 5mins | **Cook:** 10mins

Ingredients:

- ✓ 2 tablespoons of extra virgin olive oil
- ✓ 4 ripe tomatoes, chopped
- ✓ 4 eggs
- ✓ salt and pepper to taste

Directions: In a skillet or frying pan, heat the oil over medium heat. Place the tomatoes in the skillet. Cook for 3-5 minutes or until the juices begin to evaporate.

Crack the eggs into the pan. Cook until preferred consistency, but do not break the yolks. Season to taste with pepper and salt.

MAPLE BRINED AND APPLE SMOKED PORK

Serv: 12 | **Prep:** 10mins | **Cook:** 12h

Ingredients:

Brine:

- ✓ 1 gallon of cold water
- ✓ 2 cups of pure maple syrup
- ✓ 1 cup Kosher salt
- ✓ 1 pork roast
- ✓ apple wood chips

Spray:

- ✓ 3/4 cup apple cider vinegar
- ✓ 1/4 cup pure maple syrup

Directions: In a large pot, mix 2 cups maple syrup, water and salt for 2 minutes until brine is well combined. Add the pork piece to the pot. Refrigerate the pot for 3 hours.

While the pork is brining, place the wood chips in a bowl and wet them with hot water.

Drain the wood chips. Place drained wood chips in a smoker. Place the grill on top of the smoker. Take the pork from the brine and place it on the smoker. Discard the brine.

Set the smoker to 280°F (138°C). In a clean spray bottle, mix 1/4 cup maple syrup and apple cider vinegar.

In the smoker, cook the pork for 12 hours, spraying the pork with vinegar spray every 45 minutes until the internal temperature of the pork reaches 195°F (90°C). Place pork on clean cutting board. Slice or shred the pork.

MARINATED CHICKEN WITH ROSEMARY

Serv: 7| **Prep:** 24-36h | **Cook:** 1h30mins

Ingredients:

- ✓ 2 (2 to 3 pounds) whole chicken
- ✓ 2 bunches of fresh parsley, chopped
- ✓ 1 bunch of fresh thyme
- ✓ 6 tablespoons of dried rosemary
- ✓ 3 tablespoons of grated lemon peel
- ✓ 12 cloves of crushed garlic
- ✓ 3 tablespoons of ground black pepper
- ✓ 1 cup of olive oil
- ✓ 1 cup white wine

Directions: To make the marinade: In a food processor, process together wine, oil, pepper, garlic, lemon zest, rosemary, thyme and parsley. Blend until ingredients are incorporated and mixture becomes smooth.

Remove the first two wing joints of the chickens and tie them with twine so that the legs are held firmly against the bodies. Rub the marinade into both the inside of the cavity and the outside; be sure to rub a little under the skin of the breasts. Place the chickens in a glass dish, breast side up, and place the rest of the marinade on the breast and around the legs. Keep the dish covered and let marinate in the refrigerator for 24-36 hours.

Preheat the oven to 350°F (175°C). Remove chickens from marinade dish, putting away excess marinade. Place in lightly greased 9-by-13-inch baking dish and bake in prepared oven until chicken juices are clear and chickens are no longer pink, about 1.5 hours.

MEXICAN CHORIZO

Serv: 8| **Prep:** 25mins | **Cook:** 15mins

Ingredients:

- ✓ 2 pounds of boneless pork shoulder
- ✓ 1 tablespoons crushed Aleppo peppers
- ✓ 1 1/2 tablespoons of chili powder
- ✓ 4 garlic cloves, minced
- ✓ 2 teaspoons of salt
- ✓ 1 teaspoon of freshly ground black pepper
- ✓ 1/2 teaspoon of dried oregano
- ✓ 1/2 teaspoon ground cumin
- ✓ 1/4 teaspoon ground cloves
- ✓ 1/4 teaspoon ground coriander
- ✓ 1/2 cup distilled white vinegar
- ✓ 2 tbsp water
- ✓ 1 teaspoon of vegetable oil

Directions: In a bowl, place pork and add cilantro, cloves, cumin, oregano, black pepper, salt, garlic, chili powder and Aleppo pepper. Lightly stir in seasonings until well combined.

Cover the bowl and chill the meat, hopper and grinder head for 1 hour in the refrigerator.

Place a medium-sized metal bowl in a large bowl filled with ice cubes to catch the ground meat. Fit the refrigerated grinder, and then grind the meat and seasonings with a coarse chopping plate. Refrigerate the ground meat for an additional 30 minutes. Mix the water, vinegar and ground meat until well combined. Form the meat into patties, then cover and refrigerate overnight to develop the flavors.

In a heavy skillet, heat vegetable oil over medium-low heat. Pan fry the meatballs for 5-8 minutes per side, or until they are nicely browned all over and no longer pink in the center.

MOM'S PIG FEET FOR THE NEW YEAR

Serv: 4| **Prep:** 20mins | **Cook:** 2h

Ingredients:

- ✓ 8 pig's feet, divided
- ✓ 2 celery ribs, chopped
- ✓ 1 onion, chopped
- ✓ 3/4 cup white vinegar
- ✓ 2 tablespoons of red pepper flakes (optional)
- ✓ 2 tablespoons of seasoned salt
- ✓ 1 tablespoon chopped garlic
- ✓ 1 teaspoon of ground black pepper
- ✓ 2 bay leaves
- ✓ water, or as much as necessary to cover

Directions: Use cold water to wash the pork feet well and then transfer them to a Dutch oven or large pot. Add bay leaf, black pepper, garlic, seasoned salt, red pepper flakes, vinegar, onion and celery to the feet. Cover with water.

Heat to a boil, reduce heat to low and simmer for about 2 hours until the meat pulls away from the bones and is tender.

MOROCCAN CHICKEN

Serv: 6| **Prep:** 20mins | **Cook:** 1h45mins

Ingredients:

Blend of Moroccan spices:

- ✓ 1/4 cup ground cinnamon
- ✓ 1/4 cup ground cumin
- ✓ 2 tablespoons of ground turmeric
- ✓ 2 tablespoons of ground coriander
- ✓ 2 tablespoons ground ginger
- ✓ 2 tablespoons crushed dried mint
- ✓ 1 tablespoon salt
- ✓ 2 teaspoons of ground black pepper
- ✓ 1/2 cup chopped dried apricots
- ✓ 1/4 cup raisins
- ✓ 1/4 cup olive oil, or as needed
- ✓ 4 chicken thighs with bone
- ✓ 1/2 small onion, chopped
- ✓ 2 teaspoons of minced garlic
- ✓ 1 cup of chicken broth
- ✓ 1/4 cup honey
- ✓ 1/2 bunch of fresh cilantro, chopped
- ✓ 1/4 cup sliced toasted almonds

Directions: In a bowl, mix the pepper, salt, mint, ginger, cilantro, turmeric, cumin and cinnamon. Measure out 1/2 cup of the spice mixture and set aside the leftover for later use.

Boil a small pot of water. Put in the raisins and apricots, and then cook for about 5 minutes until the fruit is soft. Drain and set aside 1/2 cup of the cooking water.

In a Dutch oven or large skillet, put enough olive oil to coat the bottom, and then turn the heat up to medium. Use 1/2 cup of the spice mixture to coat the chicken and place it in the hot oil. Let it cook for 3-4 minutes on each side until it comes off the pan easily and is golden brown.

In the skillet with the chicken, stir in the garlic and onion, then cook and stir for 2-3 minutes until aromatic. Add the honey, chicken broth, and 1/2 cup of the reserved water from the fruit, raisins and apricots, then reduce the heat to low and put the lid on. Cook for 1-2 hours until the chicken becomes very soft.

Serve the chicken decorated with almonds and cilantro.

ITALIAN STYLE MUSSELS

Serv: 8 | **Prep:** 45mins | **Cook:** 10mins

Ingredients:

- ✓ 8 pounds of fresh mussels
- ✓ 1 carrot, peeled and sliced
- ✓ 1 onion, peeled and sliced
- ✓ 1 1/2 celery stalks, sliced
- ✓ 1 bay leaf
- ✓ 3 black peppercorns
- ✓ 2 lemon slices
- ✓ 1/2 bottle of white wine

Directions: To get your mussels ready, scrape off any growth or life on the outside of the shells, and remove a small bunch of beard or dark hairs that come out of the side of the shells. While you are doing this, soak them in cold water. Shells are normally unopened when you buy them.

It's okay if they open under water, shells that remain open once touched should be discarded.

This potion can be made 2 hours in advance in case the mussels are kept in a cool place. Reserve clean mussels.

Mix white wine, lemon slices, peppercorns, bay leaves, celery, onion and carrot in a large heavy-bottomed pot.

Bring to a boil over high heat, and place 1/3 of the cleaned mussels in. Put the lid on the pot and cook, shaking, every minute or so to help the mussels cook equally.

Once each mussel is open, using a slotted spoon, remove from the pot and serve. Continue to cook the rest of the mussels in the same liquid.

ORANGE CHILE TILAPIA

Serv: 2 | **Prep:** 10mins | **Cook:** 15mins

Ingredients:

- ✓ 4 (4 ounce) Tilapia fillets
- ✓ 2 tablespoons of olive oil
- ✓ 2 tablespoons of chili powder
- ✓ 1 teaspoon garlic powder
- ✓ 1 tablespoon of cayenne pepper
- ✓ 1 tablespoon ground cumin
- ✓ 1 tablespoon of grated orange peel

Directions: Preheat the oven to 350°F (175°C) ahead of time.

In a glass baking dish, lay the Tilapia and use olive oil to rub each side. In a small bowl, add cumin, cayenne pepper, and chili powder together and mix well. Use the spice mixture to dredge both sides of the Tilapia, and dredge the orange zest on top.

In the preheated oven, let the Tilapia bake for about 15 minutes until it is no longer translucent and flakes easily with a fork.

BACON MUFFINS

Serv: 9 | **Prep:** 20mins | **Cook:** 20mins

Ingredients:

- ✓ 8 strips of raw bacon, chopped
- ✓ 1/2 cup chopped onion
- ✓ 1/2 cup chopped green bell pepper
- ✓ 9 big eggs
- ✓ 3 chives, chopped, or more to taste
- ✓ coarse sea salt to taste

Directions: Begin by preheating the oven to 175°C (or 350°F). Prepare a muffin pan lined with paper.

In a medium bowl, mix the green bell pepper, onion, and bacon. Spread bacon mixture into each muffin cup, covering each cup until 3/4 full. Crack 1 egg into each cup. Add a pinch of salt and chives over each egg.

Bake for about 20 minutes in the prepared oven until the eggs are set.

PALEO SCRAMBLED EGGS

Serv: 2 | **Prep:** 5mins | **Cook:** 5mins

Ingredients:

- ✓ 4 eggs
- ✓ 1/4 cup of coconut milk
- ✓ salt and ground black pepper to taste

Directions: In a bowl, beat the eggs. Stir in the pepper, salt and coconut milk until well combined.

Prepare a skillet and heat over medium-low; add egg mixture. Cook, stirring, for 5-7 minutes until firm and fluffy.

PAN SEARED SALMON AND SCALLOPS

Serv: 8 | **Prep:** 25mins | **Cook:** 15mins

Ingredients:

- ✓ 1/2 cup unsalted macadamia nut pieces
- ✓ 1 cup packaged fresh coriander leaves
- ✓ 1/2 cup chopped green onions
- ✓ 3 tablespoons fresh chopped ginger
- ✓ 1 tablespoon chopped garlic
- ✓ 1 lemon, peeled and squeezed
- ✓ 3/4 cup macadamia nut oil or more if needed
- ✓ 4 tablespoons of olive oil
- ✓ 8 salmon fillets, with skin
- ✓ 16 large scallops
- ✓ Kosher salt to taste

Directions: Making Macadamia and Cilantro Pesto: In a blender bowl, place macadamia nut oil, lemon zest, lemon juice, garlic, ginger, green onion, cilantro and macadamia nuts. Puree until smooth, adding more oil if necessary. Then season with Kosher salt to taste.

Over medium-high heat, heat 2 very large skillets with 2 tablespoons oil in each until smoking. Add Kosher salt to season scallops and salmon to taste. Cook salmon fillets for 5 minutes until crisp and golden brown, flesh side down. Turn, cook for 5 minutes on skin side until preferred doneness. Arrange seared salmon on serving plates. Brown the scallops for 2-3 minutes on each side until golden brown.

Spread a little macadamia-cilantro pesto over the salmon to serve. Decorate with 2 pieces of seared scallops.

PAN GRILLED PORK WITH ZUCCHINI RIBBONS

Serv: 4 | **Prep:** 20mins | **Cook:** 9mins

Ingredients:

Marinade:

- ✓ 2 tablespoons of olive oil
- ✓ 2 tbsp water
- ✓ 2 tablespoons of pineapple juice
- ✓ 2 tablespoons of red wine vinegar
- ✓ 1 tablespoon sugar
- ✓ 1/2 teaspoon of onion flakes, or to taste
- ✓ 1/4 teaspoon salt
- ✓ 1/4 teaspoon garlic grains
- ✓ 1/4 teaspoon ground black pepper
- ✓ 1 pinch of ground cumin
- ✓ 1 pinch of paprika
- ✓ 1 pinch of ground coriander
- ✓ 1 pinch of ground ginger
- ✓ 3/4 pound of pork chops boned and cut in the middle

Zucchini Ribbons:

- ✓ 1 3/4 pounds of zucchini, ends cut off
- ✓ 1/4 cup butter
- ✓ 4 garlic cloves, crushed
- ✓ 1/2 teaspoon of sea salt
- ✓ 1/4 teaspoon ground black pepper
- ✓ 1 teaspoon of olive oil

Directions: In a bowl, combine ginger, cilantro, paprika, cumin, 1/4 teaspoon black pepper, garlic powder, 1/4 teaspoon salt, onion flakes, sugar, red wine vinegar, pineapple juice, water and 2 tablespoons olive oil. Place pork chops; coat completely by turning. Marinate pork chops for 1/2 hour in refrigerator.

Turn zucchini over once it gets close to the seeds; begin cutting the other side.

In a skillet, heat the butter over medium heat. Cook, stirring the garlic, for 1 minute or until fragrant. Toss in the zucchini ribbons. Add 1/4 teaspoon pepper and 1/2 teaspoon salt for seasoning; cook stirring for 2-3 minutes or until ribbons are just tender.

Over medium-high heat, heat grill pan. Brush with olive oil. Cook pork chops for 3 minutes on each side or until cooked through and golden brown. An instant-read thermometer should register at least 145°F (63°C) when inserted in the center. Arrange the pork chop next to the zucchini ribbons to serve.

PERFECT FLAT IRON STEAK

Serv: 6 | **Prep:** 15mins | **Cook:** 8mins

Ingredients:

- ✓ 1 flat iron steak
- ✓ 2 1/2 tablespoons of olive oil
- ✓ 2 garlic cloves, minced
- ✓ 1 teaspoon fresh parsley chopped
- ✓ 1/4 teaspoon fresh rosemary chopped
- ✓ 1/2 teaspoon chopped fresh chives
- ✓ 1/4 cup of Cabernet Sauvignon
- ✓ 1/2 teaspoon salt
- ✓ 3/4 teaspoon of ground black pepper
- ✓ 1/4 teaspoon dry mustard powder

Directions: Carry the steak in a large resealable bag. Combine mustard powder, pepper, salt, Cabernet, chives, rosemary, parsley, garlic and olive oil in a small bowl. Add to the bag containing the steak. Press out as much air as possible; close bag. Marinate in refrigerator for 2 to 3 hours.

Bring a nonstick skillet to medium-high heat. Fry steak, 3-4 minutes per side, in hot skillet until desired doneness is reached.

Remove the marinade. Steaks taste best when they are medium-cooked. Allow steak to rest for about 5 minutes before serving.

PERFECT ROAST CHICKEN

Serv: 6| **Prep:** 15mins | **Cook:** 2h

Ingredients:

- ✓ 1 whole chicken
- ✓ 1 cup margarine, softened
- ✓ 1 tablespoon of garlic salt
- ✓ 1 teaspoon of coarsely ground black pepper
- ✓ 1 teaspoon of dried thyme
- ✓ 1 teaspoon of dried parsley
- ✓ 1 pinch of dried rosemary

Directions: Begin by preheating the oven to 350°F (175°C).

Rinse and dry the chicken well with paper towels. In a bowl, combine the rosemary, parsley, thyme, black pepper, garlic salt and margarine; then rub the entire outside of the chicken well.

Add any remaining margarine mixture to the cavity of the chicken. Arrange the chicken in a glass-baking dish.

Bake the chicken for about 2 hours in the preheated oven until the chicken is browned and the juices come out clear.

If you insert an instant-read thermometer into the thickest part of the thigh (without touching the bone), it should reach a minimum of 70°C (160°F).

CHICKEN WITH PINEAPPLE AND CRANBERRIES

Serv: 8| **Prep:** 5mins | **Cook:** 40mins

Ingredients:

- ✓ 4 pounds of skinless, boneless chicken breast
- ✓ 1 (16 ounce) can of whole cranberry sauce
- ✓ 1 (20 oz) can crushed pineapple, drained
- ✓ 1/2 teaspoon ground cinnamon

Directions: Begin by preheating the oven to 375°F (190°C).

In a lightly oiled baking dish, place the chicken and use a fork to pierce it. Layer the chicken on top with the cranberry sauce and pineapple. Add the cinnamon.

Wrap dish; bake for 25 minutes in prepared oven. Remove lid; bake until juices are clear and chicken is cooked through, about 15 minutes longer.

CHICKEN AND CACTUS

Serv: 2| **Prep:** 10mins | **Cook:** 20mins

Ingredients:

- ✓ 2 halves of chicken breast
- ✓ 3 fresh tomatillos, without skin
- ✓ 3 fresh Jalapeno peppers, with seeds
- ✓ 1 can of canned nopales (cactus), drained

Directions: Bring a pot of water to a boil. Add chicken breasts to boiling water; cook for 10 minutes, or until juices run clear and center is no longer pink. Pierce the center with an instant-read thermometer; it should read at least 74°C/165°F. Drain and set aside to cool the chicken. Once cool enough to handle, shred into small strips.

Refill the pot with water and bring to a boil. Add the nopales, Jalapeno peppers and tomatillos to the boiling water; cook for 5 minutes, or until the vegetables are tender. Drain.

In a blender, add the jalapeno peppers and tomatillos. Blend until the mixture is smooth, and then pour into the pot with the shredded chicken. Set the pot over medium heat.

Cut the nopales into small pieces and add them to the mixture. Simmer for 5 minutes, or until mixture is fully heated through.

PACKETS OF PORK CHOPS

Serv: 2| **Prep:** 15mins | **Cook:** 45mins

Ingredients:

- ✓ 2 pork chops
- ✓ 2 large sweet potatoes
- ✓ 2 slices of onion
- ✓ 2 apples - peeled, cored and sliced

Directions: Preheat the oven to 350°F (175°C).

Lay out a sheet of aluminum foil large enough to hold the ingredients. On the foil, place the pork chops, then place the apple, onion and sweet potato on top of the chops. Fold over and seal each package.

Bake at 350°F (175°C) for 45 minutes, or until potato is soft when pricked with a fork.

(Note: Do not open the packages while baking because it will let steam escape and dry out the pork chops. Also, be careful when opening because the steam may cause burns).

PORK LOIN WITH CUMIN CRUST

Serv: 6| **Prep:** 10mins | **Cook:** 1h

Ingredients:

- ✓ 2 tablespoons of cumin seeds, crushed
- ✓ 1 teaspoon salt
- ✓ 1 teaspoon of mustard powder
- ✓ 1/2 teaspoon of dried thyme
- ✓ 1/2 teaspoon of dried oregano
- ✓ 1 tablespoon of vegetable oil
- ✓ 3 pounds of boneless pork loin roast

Directions: Preheat the oven to 165°C/325°F. To make a paste, mix the vegetable oil, oregano, thyme, mustard powder, and salt and cumin seeds in a small bowl.

Place the roast, fat side up, in the roasting pan. On the sides and top of the roast, rub in the spice mixture. Place a meat thermometer in the roast. Place in the oven.

Roast for 1 hour until internal temperature reaches 67°C/155°F. Remove from oven. Allow to rest for 15 minutes. The temperature of the roast will rise to 63°C/145°F. Cut and serve.

PORK PICADILLO

Serv: 6| **Prep:** 15mins | **Cook:** 20mins

Ingredients:

- ✓ 2 tablespoons of olive oil
- ✓ 1 onion, diced
- ✓ 2 garlic cloves, crushed
- ✓ 2 1/2 pounds of ground pork
- ✓ salt and pepper to taste
- ✓ 1 yellow bell pepper, cut into thin strips
- ✓ 1 green bell pepper, cut into thin strips

- ✓ 1 red bell pepper, cut into thin strips
- ✓ 1 1.5 oz box of raisins
- ✓ 1 bunch of spinach, chopped

Directions: In a large skillet, over medium heat, heat the olive oil. Cook by stirring the garlic and onion in the oil for about 5 minutes until tender. Remove garlic and onion from skillet; set aside. Break pork into crumbs in the skillet; cook until no longer pink. Transfer garlic and onion back to skillet; stir in pork. Sprinkle with pepper and salt. Cook with a lid on for 5 minutes. Stir raisins, yellow bell bell pepper, red bell bell pepper and green bell bell pepper into mixture; cook covered for another 5 minutes. Add spinach to skillet; stir, then serve.

FAST POLYNESIAN CHICKEN

Serv: 5 | **Prep:** mins | **Cook:** 1h

Ingredients:

- ✓ 6 chicken legs
- ✓ 1 (15.25 ounce) can of fruit cocktail

Directions: Preheat an oven to 175°C/350°F.

Rinse and dry the chicken pieces. Remove skins if desired. Place chicken in a 9x13-inch baking dish.

Spoon the fruit cocktail and juices over the chicken evenly. In preheated oven, bake for 1 hour without turning or basting. Cool and serve.

ROAST PORK CHOP

Serv: 4 | **Prep:** 10mins | **Cook:** 1h20mins

Ingredients:

- ✓ 4 pork chops cut thickly
- ✓ salt and pepper to taste

- ✓ 1 large onion, peeled and sliced
- ✓ 1 cup of water

Directions: Set the oven to 350°F (175°C) and begin preheating.

Place roasting rack in a shallow roasting pan or baking dish. Arrange the chops on the grill. Add pepper and salt to taste. Use the onion slices to cover the chops. Pour the water into the bottom of the pan, making sure it's not high enough to touch the chops. Cover with a tight-fitting lid or aluminum foil; roast for 1 hour.

To check degree of doneness, cut into chops. Once the chops are done all the way through, remove the lid or foil; transfer them back to the oven to brown slightly, 15-20 minutes. Watch carefully during the browning process.

ROASTED EGGPLANT, TOMATOES AND ZUCCHINI

Serv: 8 | **Prep:** 20mins | **Cook:** 30mins

Ingredients:

- ✓ 4 small purple eggplants
- ✓ 1 pinch of salt and freshly ground pepper to taste
- ✓ 5 Roma Tomatoes
- ✓ 2 zucchini, diced
- ✓ 1 large yellow onion, cut into cubes
- ✓ 5 garlic cloves, or more to taste, peeled
- ✓ 2 tablespoons of olive oil, or to taste

Directions: Set the oven to 450°F (230°C) for preheating. Use aluminum foil to line the rimmed baking sheet.

Place colander over a bowl. Place eggplant cubes in colander. Sprinkle the cubes generously with salt. Let them sit for 30 minutes until drained.

In a bowl, mix the garlic, zucchini, tomatoes and onion. Drizzle the mixture with olive oil. Stir the mixture until coated. Season the mixture with pepper and salt.

Wash eggplant until all salt is removed. Use a paper towel to dry eggplant. Add eggplant to tomato mixture; toss to combine. Drizzle olive oil if necessary, making sure eggplant cubes are well coated. Transfer vegetable mixture to prepared baking sheet.

Roast in preheated oven for 30 minutes until vegetables are tender.

ROASTED CAULIFLOWER STEAKS

Serv: 4 | **Prep:** 10mins | **Cook:** 35mins

Ingredients:

- ✓ 1 head of cauliflower, trimmed
- ✓ 2 tablespoons of extra virgin olive oil
- ✓ 1/4 teaspoon garlic powder
- ✓ salt and ground black pepper to taste

Directions: Set an oven to 450°F (230°C) and begin preheating. Use aluminum foil to line a baking sheet.

Place cauliflower on a cutting board, stem side up; slice vertically into about 4 slices of uniform thickness. Arrange the "steaks" on the lined baking sheet. Drizzle steaks with olive oil; season with black pepper, salt and garlic powder.

In the prepared oven, roast for 20 minutes, use a spatula to turn and continue to roast for another 15 minutes until the edges darken and the center becomes soft.

ROAST PORK LOIN

Serv: 8 | **Prep:** 20mins | **Cook:** 1h

Ingredients:

- ✓ 3 garlic cloves, minced
- ✓ 1 tablespoon of dried rosemary
- ✓ salt and pepper to taste
- ✓ 2 pounds of boneless pork loin roast
- ✓ 1/4 cup olive oil
- ✓ 1/2 cup white wine

Directions: Begin by preheating the oven to 350°F (175°C).

Mash garlic with pepper, salt and rosemary to make a paste. Use a sharp knife to pierce the meat in a few places, and then press the garlic paste into them. Rub the olive oil and remaining garlic mixture over the meat.

Place the pork loin in the oven, turn and baste with the liquids from the pan. Bake for 60 minutes or until pork is no longer pink in the center.

An instant-read thermometer should register 145°F (63°C) when inserted in the center. Discard the roast from the oven and move it to a serving platter. In the skillet, heat the wine and whisk to loosen the browned bits on the bottom.

Taste with the cooking juices.

ROAST PORK WITH ROSEMARY

Serv: 6 | **Prep:** 20mins | **Cook:** 2h

Ingredients:

- ✓ 3 pounds pork tenderloin
- ✓ 1 tablespoon olive oil
- ✓ 2 cloves garlic, minced

✓ 3 tablespoons dried rosemary

Directions: Set the oven to 375°F (190°C) and begin preheating.

Rub the tenderloin or roast liberally with olive oil and sprinkle the garlic on top. Transfer to a baking sheet, sprinkle with the rosemary.

Bake at 375°F (190°C) until the internal temperature of the pork reaches 145°F (63°C) or for 2 hours.

SALISBURY STEAK

Serv: 6| **Prep:** 20mins | **Cook:** 20mins

Ingredients:

✓ 1 can of French onion soup
✓ 1 1/2 pounds of ground beef
✓ 1/2 cup dry breadcrumbs
✓ 1 egg
✓ 1/4 teaspoon salt
✓ 1/8 teaspoon ground black pepper
✓ 1 tablespoon all-purpose flour
✓ 1/4 cup of ketchup
✓ 1/4 cup water
✓ 1 tablespoon Worcestershire sauce
✓ 1/2 teaspoon mustard powder

Directions: In a large bowl, mix together 1/3 cup condensed French onion soup with breadcrumbs, egg, black pepper, salt and ground meat. Form into 6 oval-shaped patties.

In a large skillet over medium-high heat, brown each side of patties. Discard excess fat.

Mix remaining soup and flour until smooth in a small bowl. Stir in water, mustard powder, Worcestershire sauce and ketchup. Place meat in the skillet. Cover and cook for 20 minutes, stirring occasionally.

SALT-CRUSTED COD FILLETS WITH LEMON DILL

Serv: 4| **Prep:** 20mins | **Cook:** 15mins

Ingredients:

✓ 4 Diamond Crystal® Kosher Salt containers
✓ 4 egg whites, lightly beaten
✓ 2 lemons, sliced
✓ 2 1/2 pounds cod fillets
✓ 1 tablespoon olive oil
✓ 1/2 teaspoon Diamond Crystal® Kosher Salt
✓ 1/4 teaspoon black pepper
✓ 2 bunches fresh dill

Directions: Preheat oven to 400°F (200°C).

In a large bowl, add the containers of Diamond Crystal Kosher Salt. Put in the egg whites. Mix well with two spoons or your hands until the consistency resembles wet sand.

In the bottom of a glass-baking dish, place 1/2 of the prepared salt; pat well. The salt should be about 1/2 inch thick.

On top of the salt, place lemon slices edge to edge. The fish may absorb too much salt if it really touches the salt; use the lemon slices as a flavor infuser and barrier. Reserve the excess lemon slices for serving and decorating.

Rub fish fillets with olive oil on each side, and use pepper and Diamond Crystal Kosher Salt to season well.

Arrange the fish fillets on top of the lemon slices, making sure the edges do not touch the salt base.

Arrange the dill so that it covers the fish entirely, saving a few sprigs to chop for decoration. Again, this will serve as a barrier to prevent the salt crust, because it has no skin to cover it, from absorbing salt during cooking, this also brings a bold and tangy flavor.

Add the rest of the salt mixture equally over the dill, smoothing gently. All corners should be covered; pat firmly to ensure a good seal without cracking.

Place in the center of the oven and bake for 15 minutes.

Let the fish rest for 5 minutes, and then break the sides of the salt crust with a strong knife before opening.

Halve each fillet. Serve with fresh chopped dill and leftover lemon slices.

SALTED AND BLACKENED TILAPIA

Serv: 2| **Prep:** 3mins | **Cook:** 6mins

Ingredients:

- ✓ 2 Tilapia fillets (4oz).
- ✓ 1 teaspoon Diamond Crystal® Kosher Salt
- ✓ 2 teaspoons Cajun seasoning

Directions: Use Diamond Crystal(R) Kosher Salt to lightly season one side of each Tilapia fillet. Rub both sides of fillets with Cajun seasoning.

In a skillet, heat the oil over medium-high heat.

When the oil becomes hot, carefully lay the fillets in the pan. Fry each side for 3 to 4 minutes, until the fish is nicely browned and can be easily shredded.

On a heated plate, place the Tilapia; cover with aluminum foil and let stand for a few minutes.

BACON WRAPPED ARTICHOKE HEARTS

Serv: 8| **Prep:** 20mins | **Cook:** 10mins

Ingredients:

- ✓ 8 cups peanut oil for frying
- ✓ 1 (16 ounce) can artichoke hearts in water, drained
- ✓ 1 (16 ounce) package bacon slices, cut into thirds crosswise
- ✓ 20 toothpicks

Directions: Heat a large saucepan or a deep-fryer with oil to 175 degrees C (350 degrees F).

Wrap a piece of bacon in each artichoke heart. Thread a toothpick through the end of the bacon to secure.

Place bacon-wrapped artichoke hearts in the hot oil, fry for 7 to 9 minutes until bacon is browned and crispy; Line the plate with paper towels, drain for about 5 minutes before serving.

HARISSA CHICKEN

Serv: 4| **Prep:** 20mins | **Cook:** 10mins

Ingredients:

- ✓ 2 tablespoons smoked paprika
- ✓ 2 cloves garlic, minced
- ✓ 1 teaspoon ground cumin
- ✓ 1 teaspoon caraway seeds
- ✓ 1 chipotle pepper in adobo sauce
- ✓ 1 teaspoon adobo sauce from chipotle peppers
- ✓ 4 skinless, boneless chicken breast halves
- ✓ 1 tablespoon extra-virgin olive oil
- ✓ salt and black pepper to taste

Directions: Bring adobo sauce, chipotle pepper, caraway seeds, cumin, garlic and smoked paprika into a mortar, then use the pestle to grind until it turns into a paste. Coat chicken breasts with the paste and set into a bowl; refrigerate, covered, for a minimum of 4 hours to overnight.

Prepare an outdoor grill for medium heat, and grease grill grate with a thin layer of oil.

Take chicken out of the marinade, and remove the marinade remaining. Brush olive oil all over the chicken breasts and add on pepper and salt. Grill chicken breasts for about 5 minutes each side until grill marks ingrained on the meat surface and no pink meat remains on the inside.

HEALTHY LAMB MEATBALLS

Serv: 4 **Prep.:** 20mins | **Cook:** 30mins

Ingredients:

- ✓ 1 pound ground lamb, or more to taste
- ✓ 1/2 cup shredded cabbage, or more to taste
- ✓ 1/3 cup diced onion
- ✓ 1 egg
- ✓ 1 1/4 tablespoons ground allspice
- ✓ 1 tablespoon freshly ground cardamom
- ✓ 1/4 teaspoon ground turmeric (optional)
- ✓ 1/4 teaspoon ground sumac (optional)
- ✓ salt and ground black pepper to taste

Directions: Start preheating the oven at 350°F (175°C).

In a pot of water, heat lamb to a boil, crumbling into small chunks, using a spoon, until cooked completely, for 5 to 10 minutes. Discard fat from the water by a spoon and drain water from meat.

Combine pepper, salt, sumac, turmeric, cardamom, allspice, egg, onion, cabbage, and cooked lamb in a bowl; roll to form into 1 1/2-inch balls. Put meatballs on a baking sheet.

Bake in the prepared oven until meatballs are cooked thoroughly and turn brown on the outside, for 25 to 30 minutes.

HERBED AND SPICED ROASTED BEEF TENDERLOIN

Serv: 8 | **Prep:** 20mins | **Cook:** 35mins

Ingredients:

- ✓ 2 tablespoons fresh rosemary
- ✓ 2 tablespoons fresh thyme leaves
- ✓ 2 bay leaves
- ✓ 4 cloves garlic
- ✓ 1 large shallot, peeled and quartered
- ✓ 1 tablespoon grated orange zest
- ✓ 1 tablespoon coarse salt
- ✓ 1 teaspoon freshly ground black pepper
- ✓ 1/2 teaspoon ground nutmeg
- ✓ 1/4 teaspoon ground cloves
- ✓ 2 tablespoons olive oil
- ✓ 2 beef tenderloin roasts, trimmed

Directions: Put cloves, nutmeg, pepper, salt, orange zest, shallot, garlic, bay leaves, thyme and rosemary in a food processor. While adding oil, run machine; process till smooth. Evenly spread mixture on all tenderloin's sides; put beef into big glass baking dish. Use foil to cover; refrigerate for a minimum of 6 hours.

Preheat an oven to 200°C/400°F; put tenderloins onto rack in a big roasting pan.

In preheated oven, roast beef for 35 minutes till inserted meat thermometer in middle of beef reads 140°. Remove from oven; loosely cover with foil and allow standing about 10 minutes. Cut beef; serve.

PALEO PEACH CRISP WITH COCONUT

Serv: 4 | **Prep:** 10mins | **Cook:** 30mins

Ingredients:

- ✓ 1 (16 ounce) package frozen peach slices
- ✓ 2 tablespoons coconut sugar, divided
- ✓ 1 1/2 cups almond flour
- ✓ 1/2 cup coconut flakes
- ✓ 1 teaspoon baking powder
- ✓ 1/2 teaspoon sea salt
- ✓ 3 tablespoons unsalted butter, cubed
- ✓ 1 teaspoon vanilla extract
- ✓ 1/4 cup slivered almonds
- ✓ 1 tablespoon coconut oil, melted

Directions:

Preheat an oven to 175 °C or 350 °F. In baking dish, put slices of peach.

In preheating oven, defrost the peaches for 5 minutes. Separate and scatter equally in baking dish. Scatter a tablespoon of sugar over.

In food processor, mix salt, baking powder, coconut flakes, almond flour and leftover 1 tablespoon of coconut sugar; pulse approximately five times till blended. Put the vanilla extract and butter; pulse several more times till crumbly. Put on top of peaches.

On top of flour mixture, spread slivered almonds. Drizzle top with coconut oil.

In prepped oven, bake for 22 to 25 minutes till golden brown.

ROASTED LEMON HERB CHICKEN

Serv: 8 | **Prep:** 15mins | **Cook:** 1h30mins

Ingredients:

- ✓ 2 teaspoons Italian seasoning
- ✓ 1/2 teaspoon seasoning salt
- ✓ 1/2 teaspoon mustard powder
- ✓ 1 teaspoon garlic powder
- ✓ 1/2 teaspoon ground black pepper
- ✓ 1 (3 pound) whole chicken
- ✓ 2 lemons
- ✓ 2 tablespoons olive oil

Directions:

Start preheating the oven at 350°F (175°C).

Mix black pepper, garlic powder, mustard powder, salt, and seasoning; put aside. Wash the chicken thoroughly, and then remove the giblets. In a 9x13-inch baking dish, place the chicken. Scatter 1 1/2 teaspoons of the spice mixture inside the chicken. Rub the leftover mixture on the outside of the chicken.

Squeeze the juice from 2 lemons into a small bowl or cup and combine with olive oil. Sprinkle the oil-juice mixture over the chicken.

Bake in the prepared oven for 1 1/2 hours until juices run clear, basting several times with the remaining oil mixture.

ROASTED PEPPERS WITH PINE NUTS AND PARSLEY

Serv: 10 | **Prep:** 20mins | **Cook:** 15mins

Ingredients:

- ✓ 2 red bell peppers
- ✓ 2 yellow bell peppers
- ✓ 2 ounces pine nuts
- ✓ 1/3 cup golden raisins
- ✓ 1 clove garlic, minced
- ✓ 1/2 cup chopped fresh parsley
- ✓ 1/2 cup olive oil

✓ salt and ground black pepper to taste

Directions: Start preheating the oven broiler; put the oven rack at about 6 inches away from the heat source. Use aluminum foil to line a baking sheet. Use a knife to separate peppers in half from top to bottom; remove the ribs, seeds and stem, then on a prepared baking sheets, place the peppers cut sides down. Cook in the oven broiler for about 10 minutes until the peppers skin turn blistered and blackened. In a bowl, place in blackened peppers and cover tightly with plastic wrap. Allow to steam for about 20 minutes while cooling down. When cool, remove and throw away the skin.

In a small dry skillet, toast pine nuts over medium-low heat, swirl the pine nuts for 1 to 2 minutes until they have nutty scent and turn to light tan color. Remove from the heat; pour into a small bowl in order to avoid overcooking.

Cut the roasted peppers into strips, and on a serving platter, place peppers strips decoratively by alternating yellow and red ones. Sprinkle peppers with parsley, garlic, raisins and toasted pine nuts. Add in olive oil in a drizzle; put salt and black pepper to season.

RONALDO'S BEEF CARNITAS

Serv: 8| **Prep:** 20mins | **Cook:** 1h

Ingredients:

✓ 4 pounds chuck roast
✓ 1 (4 ounce) green chile peppers, chopped
✓ 2 tablespoons chili powder
✓ 1/2 teaspoon dried oregano
✓ 1/2 teaspoon ground cumin
✓ 2 cloves garlic, minced

✓ salt to taste

Directions: Set the oven to 150°C or 300°F to preheat.

On a heavy foil that is big enough to enclose the meat, position the roast. Mix together garlic, salt to taste, cumin, oregano, chili powder and green chile peppers in a small bowl. Mix well and rub the spice mixture over the meat.

Wrap the meat entirely in foil and put in a roasting pan.

Bake at 150°C or 300°F until the roast just falls apart using a fork, about 3 1/2-4 hours. Take out of the oven and use 2 forks to shred the meat.

ROSEMARY FRITTATA

Serv: 8| **Prep:** 20mins | **Cook:** 25mins

Ingredients:

✓ 3 tablespoons olive oil
✓ 1 small red onion, chopped
✓ 3 cloves garlic, chopped
✓ 2 green bell peppers, diced
✓ 12 eggs, beaten
✓ 1/2 cup chopped fresh basil leaves
✓ 4 sprigs fresh rosemary, leaves removed and chopped
✓ 1 teaspoon salt
✓ 1/2 teaspoon freshly ground black pepper
✓ 1 cup olive oil for frying
✓ 1 sweet potato, peeled and cut into thin matchsticks

Directions: Set oven to 350°F (175°C) to preheat.

In an ovenproof skillet, heat 3 tablespoons olive oil over medium heat. Add garlic and onion; stir-fry for about 5 minutes until translucent. Mix in green peppers, and continue to cook and stir for 5 more minutes until they start to become tender. Pour eggs over vegetable mixture, and mix in pepper, salt, rosemary, and basil. Turn heat down to medium-low, and allow eggs to stand over the heat for about 10 minutes or until the eggs start to set.

Move the skillet to the preheated oven and bake for 15 minutes until the frittata is completely firm.

Meanwhile, in a large saucepan or deep fryer, heat 1-cup olive oil to 375°F (190°C). Deep-fry the sweet potatoes slices, 1 layer at a time, for about 5 minutes until they are crispy and golden brown. Take potato slices out of the pan using a slotted spoon and allow draining on paper towels. Put fried sweet potato slices on top of baked frittata and serve right away.

TUNISIAN FRIED PEPPERS & EGGS

Serv: 4 | **Prep:** 20mins | **Cook:** 15mins

Ingredients:

- ✓ 4 cloves garlic, diced
- ✓ 1 tablespoon caraway seeds
- ✓ 1 pinch salt
- ✓ 3 tablespoons olive oil
- ✓ 2/3 cup mild chile peppers, chopped
- ✓ 1 1/2 cups green bell peppers, seeded and chopped
- ✓ 2 cups tomatoes, seeded and chopped
- ✓ 4 eggs
- ✓ salt and ground black pepper to taste

Directions: Against a mixing bowl's side/in a mortar and pestle, mash pinch of salt, caraway seeds and garlic.

In a skillet, heat 1 tbsp. olive oil on medium heat. Mix chile peppers in. Stir and cook for 5

minutes till peppers are soft. Take out of skillet. Put aside. Put another tbsp. oil into skillet. Cook tomatoes and bell peppers for 5 minutes more till tomatoes start to break down and peppers are soft. Add bell-tomato pepper mixture into hot peppers. Mix caraway seeds and mashed garlic in. On serving platter/plates, spoon veggies on.

In skillet, heat leftover oil. Fry eggs till yolks are to preferred consistency and whites are set. 4-5 minutes for fully set yolks and 2-3 minutes for runny yolks. On veggie mixture, put fried eggs. Season with pepper and salt to taste.

THAI STYLE SHRIMP

Serv: 4 | **Prep:** 10mins | **Cook:** 20mins

Ingredients:

- ✓ 4 cloves garlic, peeled
- ✓ 1 (1 inch) piece fresh ginger root
- ✓ 1 fresh jalapeno pepper, seeded
- ✓ 1/2 teaspoon salt
- ✓ 1/2 teaspoon ground turmeric
- ✓ 2 tablespoons vegetable oil
- ✓ 1 medium onion, diced
- ✓ 1 pound medium shrimp - peeled and deveined
- ✓ 2 tomatoes, seeded and diced
- ✓ 1 cup coconut milk
- ✓ 3 tablespoons chopped fresh basil leaves

Directions: In the container of a blender or food processor, mix turmeric, salt, jalapeno, ginger and garlic and then process to form a smooth paste. Reserve.

Over medium heat, heat oil in a skillet and then add onion. Cook while stirring often until translucent. Stir in spice paste and then cook for several minutes to release the oils.

Place in shrimp and let to cook for several minutes until turns pink. Add coconut milk and tomatoes. Cover and let simmer for around five minutes. Uncover and simmer for 5 more minutes to thicken the sauce. Mix in fresh basil during the final minute of cooking

WHOLE30® COCONUT CHICKEN CURRY

Serv: 8 | **Prep:** 25mins | **Cook:** 1h30mins

Ingredients:

- ✓ 3 tablespoons coconut oil
- ✓ 1 1/2 pounds skinless, boneless chicken breast halves, cubed
- ✓ 2 onions, sliced
- ✓ 1 red bell pepper, sliced
- ✓ 1 jalapeno pepper, seeded and minced
- ✓ 4 small garlic cloves, minced
- ✓ 1 (1 inch) piece fresh ginger, peeled and minced
- ✓ 1 large sweet potato, peeled and cubed
- ✓ 1 green plantain, sliced into 1/2-inch rounds and quartered
- ✓ 3 small carrots, peeled and sliced into rounds
- ✓ 2 (14 ounce) cans coconut milk, shaken
- ✓ 1 (24 ounce) container crushed tomatoes
- ✓ 1/2 cup water
- ✓ 1 cup packed baby kale
- ✓ 3 tablespoons curry powder, or more to taste
- ✓ 1 tablespoon sea salt
- ✓ 1 tablespoon ground black pepper
- ✓ 1 1/2 teaspoons dried cilantro

Directions: In a heavy bottomed frying pan, heat the coconut oil on medium-low heat, until it shimmers. Add the chicken and let it cook for about 7 minutes, tossing to prevent it from burning and sticking, until it has no

visible pink color in the middle. Transfer the chicken to a bowl.

In the frying pan, mix the ginger, garlic, jalapeno pepper, red bell pepper and onions. Cook and stir for around 7 minutes, until the vegetables become soft. Add the carrots, plantain and sweet potato and cook for around 5 minutes, stirring from time to time, until they become a bit tender.

Pour the water, tomatoes and coconut milk into the vegetable mixture, then mix to blend. Let cook for around 30 minutes with a cover, until the flavors combine. Add the cilantro, black pepper, salt, curry powder, kale, and let cook for around 30 more minutes, until the carrots and sweet potatoes become soft.

GINGER AND LIME SALMON

Serv: 6 | **Prep:** 15mins | **Cook:** 15mins

Ingredients:

- ✓ 1 (1 1/2-pound) salmon fillet
- ✓ 1 tablespoon olive oil
- ✓ 1 teaspoon seafood seasoning (such as Old Bay®)
- ✓ 1 teaspoon ground black pepper
- ✓ 1 (1 inch) piece fresh ginger root, peeled and thinly sliced
- ✓ 6 cloves garlic, minced
- ✓ 1 lime, thinly sliced

Directions: Position oven rack approximately 6 to 8 inches away from the heat source and preheat broiler; set oven's broiler to Low setting if there is. Line aluminum foil over a baking sheet.

Arrange salmon on the prepared baking sheet, skin side down; rub olive oil over the salmon. Season fish with black pepper and seafood seasoning. Place ginger slices on top of salmon and scatter garlic over. Arrange lime slices over ginger-garlic layer.

Broil salmon for about 10 minutes until heated through and starting to turn opaque; watch carefully. Turn broiler to high setting if there is; keep broiling for 5 to 10 minutes longer or until salmon is thoroughly cooked and easily flaked using a fork.

STUCK'S KOSHER DILLS

Serv: 8 | **Prep:** 15mins | **Cook:** 20mins

Ingredients:

- ✓ 3 cups water
- ✓ 1 cup distilled white vinegar
- ✓ 1/4 cup salt
- ✓ 2 cloves garlic, or more to taste
- ✓ 2 sprigs fresh dill, or more to taste
- ✓ 3 small cucumbers, or to taste
- ✓ 3 (1 pint) canning jars with lids and rings

Directions: Boil salt, vinegar and water in a saucepan; cook for 2-3 minutes till salt melts.

Sterilize the lids and jars for at least 5 minutes in boiling water. Pack garlic, dill and cucumbers in sterilized, hot jars. Put vinegar mixture over; fill to within 1/4-in. from the top. Run a thin spatula/knife to remove any air bubbles around jar's insides after filling them. Use a moist paper towel to wipe the jar rims to remove any food residue. Put lids over; screw on rings.

Put a rack on the bottom of a big stockpot; use water to fill halfway. Boil; use a holder to lower the jars in boiling water, leave a 2-in. space between the jars. If needed, add more boiling water so water level is at least 1-in. above jar tops; put water on a rolling boil and cover the pot. Process for 15 minutes.

Take the jars from the stockpot; put on a wood/cloth-covered surface till cool, a few inches apart. Use a finger to press top of every lid when cool to be sure the seal is tight and lid does not move down or up at all; keep for 1 month minimum in a dark, cool area.

GRILLED BEEF TENDERLOIN

Serv: 8 | **Prep:** 30mins | **Cook:** 55mins

Ingredients:

- ✓ 1 (5 pound) whole beef tenderloin
- ✓ 6 tablespoons olive oil
- ✓ 8 large garlic cloves, minced
- ✓ 2 tablespoons minced fresh rosemary
- ✓ 1 tablespoon dried thyme leaves
- ✓ 2 tablespoons coarsely ground black pepper
- ✓ 1 tablespoon salt

Directions: To prepare the beef: Use a sharp knife to remove excess fat. For the thin tip end, fold under to about the thickness of the rest of the roast. Use butcher's twine to bind and continue to tie the roast with the twine every 1 1/2-2-in. (this can help the roast maintain its shape). Use scissors to snip the silver skin to make sure the roast does not bow while cooking. Combine salt, pepper, thyme, rosemary, garlic, and oil; rub this mixture over the roast until coated. Put the meat aside.

Set all gas burners on high for 10 minutes or build a charcoal fire in half the grill. Use tongs to lubricate the grate with a rag soaked with oil. On the hot rack, arrange the beef and grill, covered, for about 5 minutes until thoroughly seared. Flip the meat and grill, covered, for another 5 minutes until the second side has thoroughly seared.

Transfer the meat to the cool side of the charcoal grill, or turn off the burner directly beneath the meat and set the other 1 or 2 burners (depending on the grill style) to medium. Cook for 45-60 minutes until a meat thermometer reaches 130° for rosy pink when you insert one into the thickest part, depending on the grill and the size of the tenderloin. Allow the meat to sit for 15 minutes before carving.

GRILLED CASSAVA FLOUR PIZZA CRUST

Serv: 4 | **Prep:** 15mins | **Cook:** 7mins

Ingredients:

- ✓ coconut oil cooking spray
- ✓ 3/4 cup lukewarm water
- ✓ 3/4 teaspoon coconut sugar
- ✓ 3/4 teaspoon active dry yeast
- ✓ 1 1/2 teaspoons avocado oil (such as Chosen Foods®)
- ✓ 1/2 teaspoon salt
- ✓ 1/4 teaspoon Italian seasoning (optional)
- ✓ 2/3 cup cassava flour (such as Otto's®), or more as needed
- ✓ 1/4 cup arrowroot powder
- ✓ 3/4 teaspoon gelatin

Directions: Preheat grill on medium heat the grease grate lightly.

Mix yeast, coconut sugar, and water until well combined in a measuring cup. Let stand for 5 minutes until it starts to create a creamy foam and yeast softens. Add Italian seasoning, salt, and avocado oil then mix well.

Mix gelatin, arrowroot powder, and cassava flour in a bowl. Place in the yeast mixture. Mix using a wooden spoon until incorporated. Add extra cassava flour, as needed, a tablespoon at a time, until you form a dough.

Cut dough to 4 even portions. Knead it and form to balls. Dust a sheet of parchment paper using arrowroot powder. Put a dough ball on it and dust the top generously. Cover it with another sheet of parchment paper. Roll to a pizza crust that is 4 inches. Repeat this with the rest of the dough balls.

Take out the top parchment paper. Grease the top of every crush using coconut-cooking spray. Turn it over and put crusts on the grill with the greased side down. Cook for 7 minutes until golden brown

CONCLUSION

Thank you again for reading **"Paleo Diet Cookbook!"**. I hope you enjoyed reading my book!

Now all you have to do is try making the recipes you like best.

Our health depends on the quality of our foods and the PALEO DIET will help you get your energy and health back!

The opinions on the paleo diet collected tell us, in a broader sense, that mechanically following a list of food trends in which foods are classified into "good" and "bad" or "allowed" and "forbidden", is a wrong approach at the base. Science has not confirmed reasons to exclude dairy, legumes and grains from one's diet (except in cases of allergies or intolerances).

<u>Get a consultation with a nutritionist to find out what diet is best for you.</u>

Good luck!

9 781914 561085